I0766506

Preface

This book is dedicated to Carrie Ann Ackerman BSN who convinced me that proper nutrition is the key to good health. As a result of good health, nutrition can also affect both some neuropathic pain as well as some inflammatory pain by decreasing the overall pain intensity of many pain syndromes. The first half of this book addresses pain physiology and describes the different types of pain while the second half of the book addresses nutrition as a means of decreasing a patient's pain.

TABLE OF CONTENTS

PAIN OVERVIEW

Pain is a defining feature for many disease diagnoses. It can serve as an index of the severity and activity of an underlying condition, a prognostic indicator, and a determinant of health service use. The International Association for the Study of Pain and the World Health Organization define pain as "an unpleasant sensory and emotional experience associated with actual or potential tissue damage or described in terms of such damage.

Approximately 20 percent of U.S. adults have chronic pain and eight percent have high-impact chronic pain meaning that the patient's pain limited at least one major life activity in 2016. Health economists from Johns Hopkins University writing in The Journal of Pain previously reported the annual cost of chronic pain is as high as $635 billion a year, which is more than the yearly costs for cancer, heart disease and diabetes. Previous studies have not shown a comprehensive analysis of the impact on health care and labor markets associated with people with chronic pain. The Johns Hopkins researchers estimated the annual economic costs of chronic pain in the U.S. by assessing incremental costs of health care due to pain and the indirect costs of pain from lower productivity. They compared the costs of health care for persons with chronic pain with those who do not report chronic pain.

Previous studies in the United States showed that mean yearly pain treatment health care expenditures for adults were $4,475. Prevalence estimates for pain conditions were 10 percent for moderate pain, 11 percent for severe pain, 33 percent for joint pain, 25 percent for arthritis, and 12 percent for functional disability. Persons with moderate pain had health care expenditures $4,516 higher than someone with no pain, and individuals with severe pain had costs $3,210 higher than those with moderate pain. Similar differences were found for other pain conditions: $4,048 higher for joint pain, $5,838 for arthritis, and $9,680 for functional disabilities. Based on the analysis of the collected data, it was previously determined that that the total cost for pain treatments in the United States ranged from $560 to $635 billion. Total incremental costs of health care due to pain ranged from $261 to $300 billion, and the value of lost productivity ranged from $299 to $334 billion. Compared with other major disease conditions, the per-person cost of pain is lower, but the total cost is higher. The scope and severity of such pain can shift widely by an individual. Because pain symptoms etiologies and the conditions vary, there is no uniform treatment to help provide patient comfort.

Decades ago, pharmaceutical companies assured health care providers that prescribing opioid medication for chronic pain wouldn't lead to addiction. The National Institute on Drug Addiction recognized that this subsequently led to a widespread misuse of prescribed opioid drugs. Now there is an opioid crisis and chronic pain patients are suffering because in many instances they are unable to get their necessary treatments because of Federal government and insurance company regulations. One solution to this problem is to develop a new pain management treatment and in order to accomplish this endeavor, pain management providers may want to investigate the analgesic effects of nutrition.

Pain anywhere in the human body is ultimately identified by a specific area in the patient's brain. Pain impulses come from a patient's site of tissue injury and are transmitted to the spinal cord and ultimately to the patient's brain where a patient's pain is perceived. The spinal cord can modulate and decrease a patient's pain by decreasing the number of pain impulses that travel to the brain, but frequently pain-relieving modalities (medications, injections etc.) are medically necessary to provide some relief. Physical, and occupational medicine as well as chiropractor therapies may decrease chronic pain symptoms. Nutrition, surgery and implantable devices and/or drugs may decrease pain as well.

There are different types of pain. Pain can be neuropathic, nociceptive or inflammatory. The pain pathway from the site of origin involves transduction (the pain stimulus is converted to an electrical charge at the nerve ending), conduction (the electrical charge travels to the spinal cord), transmission (the pain impulse goes to the brain through the spinal cord) and then the pain is perceived by the brain. The biochemical mediators of pain transmission are prostaglandins, leukotrienes, substance P, histamine, bradykinin and serotonin.

There are essentially two types of pain transmission fibers. 1. A-delta fibers which involve small receptive fields, and are thermal and mechanical receptors, are myelinated and are rapidly conducting (10-30 m/sec) and have large diameters. 2. C-fibers which have broad receptive fields, and are polymodal, are unmyelinated, slower conducting (.5-2.0 m/sec) and have small diameters. These fibers ascend to the patient's brain where a patient perceives pain. There are also descending inhibitory tracts in the spinal cord that can decrease painful impulses that are traveling to the brain from the site of the origin of the pain. Persistent pain impulses to the spinal cord and brain can become permanent which results in a chronic pain syndrome. Hyperalgesia is a lowered threshold to different types of noxious stimuli. Allodynia is a painful response to what should normally be non-painful stimuli.

The transduction (formation of a pain impulse) can be decreased by non-steroidal anti-inflammatory drugs (NSAIDs such as ibuprophen), antihistamines, membrane stabilizing agents, local anesthetic cream, opioids, bradykinin and serotonin antagonists. Transmission and modulation of painful impulses are decreased by spinal opioids, alpha 2 agonists, NMDA receptor antagonists, NSAIDs, nociceptive inhibitors and potassium channel openers. In chronic pain states, connections between neurons, properties of neurotransmitters, receptors and ion channels are affected which ultimately decreases the body's pain inhibitory systems (which causes increased pain). Injury, inflammation, and disease are the perpetrators of pain stimuli which can produce permanent nervous system changes and are pivotal to the development of hypersensitivity of inflammatory pain and ultimately enables the nervous system to modify its function according to different conditions or demands placed upon it.

The chronic pain treatment armamentarium includes nonopioids (acetaminophen, NSAIDs and COX-2 inhibitors like Celebrex), opioids (mu-opioid agonists, mixed agonist-antagonists), adjuvant analgesics, antidepressants, anticonvulsants, topical agents/local anesthetics and nutrition. Nonopioids: include acetaminophen which inhibits prostaglandin production in the central nervous system (CNS). This drug has no effect on blocking peripheral prostaglandin production and no anti-inflammatory or antirheumatic activity.

NSAIDS are used to decrease both acute and chronic pain. These drugs include acetylated (aspirin) and nonacetylated (diflunisal), acetic acid (diclofenac); propionic acid (naproxen); fenamic acid (mefenamic acid); enolic acids (piroxicam); nonacidic (nabumetone); ibuprofen, and selective COX-2s (celecoxib). The mechanism of action is to exhibit both peripheral and central effects; anti-inflammatory and analgesic effects, inhibition of cyclooxygenase and prostaglandin production and inhibition of leukotriene B4 production and lipoxins (signaling resolution of inflammation).

Opioid drugs can be addicting and include morphine, hydromorphone, fentanyl, oxycodone, oxymorphone, meperidine, codeine, methadone, tramadol etc. The opioid mechanism of action in the body includes binding to opioid receptors in the central nervous system (CNS) to inhibit transmission of nociceptive (pain) input from the periphery of the body to the spinal cord, and causes activation of descending pathways that modulate transmission in the spinal cord and results in alteration of the limbic system activity and modifies sensory and affective pain aspects.

Tricyclic antidepressant medications include amitriptyline, desipramine, doxepin, imipramine and nortriptyline. The Mechanism of action of these drugs is a reduction in the action potential firing of sodium channel activity, the Inhibition of reuptake of NE and 5-HT and the analgesia is independent of antidepressant function. SSRIs (Selective Serotonin Reuptake Inhibitors) selectively inhibit 5-HT reuptake without affecting NE. Examples include citalopram, fluoxetine, fluvoxamine, paroxetine, and sertraline. The mechanism of action of these drugs does not affect pain transmission. Therefore, no pain relief is expected.

SNRIs (Serotonin/Noradrenaline Reuptake Inhibitors) include duloxetine, milnacipran, and venlafaxine. The mechanism of action of these drugs is to block the reuptake of

5-HT and sodium and is better tolerated and have a lower tendency for drug-drug interactions, and better overdose safety and do provide pain relief in some patients.

Spasmolytic drugs enhance the level of pain inhibition by mimicking or enhancing the actions of endogenous inhibitory substances, such as GABA, reducing the level of nerve excitation. This activity ultimately decreases muscle the muscle spasms which may cause pain. Common examples are cyclobenzaprine, methocarbamol, carisoprodol, tizanidine, baclofen and orphenadrine (diphenhydramine). Usual adverse effects that may occur if the dosage is too high are sedation, lethargy & confusion (cyclobenzaprine) and dependence (carisoprodol).

Topical analgesic medications include lidocaine patches 5% and eutectic mixtures of lidocaine and prilocaine as well as capsaicin cream/patches or diclofenac cream/liquid/gel/patches. The mechanism of action of topical anesthetics are to block sodium channels and inhibit generation of abnormal impulses by damaged nerves and to inhibit substance P release from sensory nerve endings and to target local inflammatory responses. This pharmacologic action ultimately keeps pain impulses from reaching a patient's brain.

Antiepileptics are drugs which suppress neuronal hyperexcitability via by reducing the neuronal influx of sodium (Na+) and calcium (Ca+ +) by direct or indirect enhancement of GABA inhibitory effects and reduce the activity of glutamate and/or blocking NMDA receptors. Examples include gabapentin, pregabalin, carbamazepine, phenytoin, divalproex sodium, clonazepam, levetiracetam, topiramate, and lamotrigine.

Decades ago, pharmaceutical companies assured health care providers that prescribing opioid medication for chronic pain wouldn't lead to addiction. The National Institute on Drug Addiction recognized that this information was false and subsequently led to a widespread misuse of prescribed opioid drugs and consequently the Federal Government declared an opioid crisis in the United States as a result of the drug companies false information.

Yellow pages and television pain treatment advertisements from pain clinics currently are multiple, and these pain providers offer various pain management treatments which will remedy a patient's pain and suffering. As a board certified anesthesiologist and pain management fellowship trained management specialist who has been a director of a pain management university hospital center and has published over 130 scientific research papers and has presented his research at national and international pain treatment meetings, I can assure readers of this book that there is not a single regimen that can totally alleviate chronic pain. Opioid therapy is frequently prescribed to pain patients because most treatments are ineffective, and this has resulted in an opioid crisis in the United States as previously mentioned.

A possible solution to this problem is nutrition. The effect of nutrition and pain reduction has been increasing in the scientific literature for the past five-ten years. This book hopefully will encourage practitioners treating chronic pain as well as patients suffering from pain to include nutrition and or a dietician in his or her chronic pain treatment. It is also hoped that pain patients themselves will research the effects of nutrition on acute and chronic pain.

References

1. Darrell J. Gaskin, Patrick Richard. The Economic Costs of Pain in the United States. The Journal of Pain, *2012*; 13 (8): 715 DOI: 10.1016/j.jpain.2012.03.009

2. Dagenais S, Caro J, Haldeman S. A systematic review of low back pain cost of illness studies in the United States and internationally. Spine J 2008; 8:8–20.

3. Dahlhamer J, Lucas J, Zelaya C, Nahin R, Mackey S, DeBar L, Kerns R, Von Korff M, Porter L, Helmick C. Prevalence of chronic pain and high impact chronic pain among adults – United States, 2016. *MMWR*. September 14, 2018.

2. PAIN EPIDEMIOLOGY

Epidemiology is the study of the distribution and determinants of health-related states or events in specified populations and the applications of this study to control health problems. Good epidemiological research on chronic pain provides important information on prevalence and factors associated with its onset and persistence. Improving our understanding of associated factors will inform our clinical management, limiting severity, and minimizing disability. In addition to a female preponderance for chronic pain, women consistently report lower pain thresholds, lower pain tolerance, and greater unpleasantness (or intensity) with pain with different analgesic sensitivity. There is some evidence for a biological basis for apparent sex differences in pain experiences involving estrogens. However, the greatest gender differences are seen in the prevalence of chronic pain syndromes. Recent evidence suggests that the occurrence of disabling chronic pain continues to rise with old age. Although the onset of pain per se does not have a clear relationship with age, there is generally a higher prevalence of chronic pain in older age.

Given that the world's population aged over 65 is likely to double in the next 40 years, treatment needs to take cognizance of pain-related co-morbidities and polypharmacy. Population-based studies of chronic pain have consistently shown that chronic pain occurrence is inversely related to socio-economic status with evidence that people living in adverse socioeconomic circumstances experience more chronic pain and greater pain severity, independent of other demographic, and clinical factors. There is also evidence of both geographical and cultural variation in occurrence of chronic pain. The occurrence of pain, or the extent to which pain interferes with life, can be influenced by demands, expectations, control and fear of re-injury at work, specific occupational factors, employer and co-worker reactions to pain, or even by broader issues such as the job market.

 There is a growing body of literature that pain is more common among people who report a history of abuse and violence at any age, in both domestic and public settings. This effect appears to be additional to the risk caused by physical injuries and pain and highlights the need to elicit any history of domestic, sexual, or criminal violence in assessing the propensity to chronic pain and in managing its impact. A prospective population-based study in the North of England concluded that there was a strong relationship between lack of sunshine, lower temperatures, and pain reporting, postulating climate as a possible risk factor. However, this relationship may be, at least in part, mediated through lifestyle factors associated with cooler and duller days (less exercise, poorer sleep, and higher reported boredom). Similarly, a seasonal effect suggests the potential role of vitamin D, low levels of which in some (but not all) studies have been shown to be related to the report of pain. Chronic pain is more than just a comorbidity of other identifiable diseases or injury. Chronic pain is acknowledged as a condition with its own agreed set of definitions and taxonomy.

The International Association for the Study of Pain (IASP) has characterized chronic pain as "pain which has persisted beyond normal tissue healing. time," which, "in the absence of other criteria," is taken to be 3 months. However, some signs of chronic pain are evidenced well before 3 months. The IASP definition of chronic pain includes pain of any severity and is not specific to a particular diagnosis or body site. The difference between acute and chronic pain is more than just duration. A more specific definition of chronic pain should also include a measure of the significance or impact of pain on daily activities. Prevalence estimates of severe disabling chronic pain lie between 5% and 15%. Although chronic pain in an individual may have a single primary cause (e.g., trauma or herpes zoster), there are other factors that influence the duration, intensity, and spectrum (physical, psychological, social, and emotional) of these effects.

Approximately 20% of the adult European population have chronic pain and, in addition to the physical and emotional burden it brings, the financial cost to society is huge, currently estimated at more than €200 billion per annum in Europe and $150 billion per annum in the USA. Fewer than 2% of sufferers ever attend a pain clinic with the remainder managed mainly in primary care, if anywhere. While important recent advances in understanding pain mechanisms bring the possibility of new treatments, management of chronic pain is nonetheless generally unsatisfactory; two-thirds of sufferers' report dissatisfaction with current treatment and most chronic pain persists for many years. We need to understand the reasons for this, with a view to improving treatment. In addition to research on the pathophysiology of pain mechanisms, it is important to understand the risk factors associated with the presence and development of chronic pain, as this will allow the design and targeting of preventive and management strategies.

The risk factors for chronic pain include socio-demographic, clinical, psychological, and biological factors, and recent research has elucidated many of these, with potential clinical relevance. One important aspect is the translation of research on risk factors from animal or small human samples to the general population. The more severe the acute pain, and the greater the number of pain sites, the more likely it is that severe chronic pain will develop. In these individuals. Anxiety, depression, and catastrophizing beliefs about pain are associated with a poorer prognosis in people with various chronic pain conditions. The prevalence of chronic pain is higher in those with other chronic diseases than those without. For example, up to a third of people with coronary heart disease also have chronic pain, and a similar percentage of people with chronic obstructive pulmonary disease have chronic pain. Individuals who were not able to work due to illness or disability were more likely to report chronic pain than those who were employed. Chronic pain syndromes generally have a higher prevalence in women with more women than men seeking treatment for it.

Consistent gender specific pain causation themes emerge, and women are found to have lower pain thresholds, experience greater unpleasantness (or intensity) with pain, and have different analgesic sensitivity. The onset of pain interfering with daily activities has been shown to be associated with neighborhood deprivation, low levels of education, and (perceived) income inequalities. Between 10% and 30% of patients undergoing common surgical procedures report persistent or intermittent pain of varying severity at 1-year postoperatively with higher rates (>40%) after major thoracic surgery and breast cancer surgery. The most studied gene in relation to pain is catechol-O-methyltransferase (COMT), an enzyme that degrades neurotransmitters including dopamine. In addition to a female preponderance for chronic pain, women consistently report lower pain thresholds, lower pain tolerance, and greater unpleasantness (or intensity) with pain with different analgesic sensitivity.

There is some evidence for a biological basis for apparent sex differences in pain experiences involving estrogens. However, the greatest gender differences are seen in the prevalence of chronic pain syndromes. Recent evidence suggests that the occurrence of disabling chronic pain continues to increase with older age. Although the onset of pain per se does not have a clear relationship with age, there is generally a higher prevalence of chronic pain in older patients.

Given that the world's population aged greater than 65 is likely to double in the next 40 years, pain treatment needs to take cognizance of pain-related co-morbidities and polypharmacy. Population-based studies of chronic pain have consistently shown that chronic pain occurrence is inversely related to socio-economic status with evidence that people living in adverse socioeconomic circumstances experience more chronic pain and greater pain severity, independent of other demographic, and clinical factors. There is also evidence of both geographical and cultural variation in occurrence of chronic pain. The occurrence of pain, or the extent to which pain interferes with life, can be influenced by demands, expectations, control and fear of re-injury at work, specific occupational factors, employer and co-worker reactions to pain, or even by broader issues such as the job market. There is a growing body of literature from large-scale national surveys that pain is more common among people who report a history of abuse and violence at any age, in both domestic and public settings. This effect appears to be additional to the risk caused by physical injuries and pain and highlights the need to elicit any history of domestic, sexual, or criminal violence in assessing the propensity to chronic pain and in managing its impact.

A prospective population-based study in the North of England concluded that there was a strong relationship between lack of sunshine, lower temperatures, and pain reporting, postulating climate as a possible risk factor. However, this relationship may be, at least in part, mediated through lifestyle factors associated with cooler and duller days (less exercise, poorer sleep, and higher reported boredom). Similarly, a seasonal effect suggests the potential role of vitamin D, low levels of which in some studies have been shown to be related to the report of pain. Although many of these risk factors are unmodifiable or not amenable to medical intervention, it is important to recognize them, as they inform a targeted approach to chronic pain assessment and management. Dedicated coding and inclusion within routinely collected data sources and disease registries will enable routine population and health system surveillance of chronic pain. This will also aid visibility, linking chronic pain to existing (better-funded) health priority areas such as cancer, injury, obesity, and healthy ageing. The existence of both individual-level risk factors and population-level risk factors for the onset or persistence of pain suggests that opportunities for intervention exist at more than one level.

Ignoring population-level factors and intervening exclusively on high-risk individuals (such as in specialist pain clinics) could limit options for reducing the overall community burden of chronic pain.

Perhaps the most important clinical factor for chronic pain at a specific site is pain (acute pain, or chronic pain at a different site). The more severe the pain and the greater number of pain sites, the more likely severe chronic pain is appreciated. This highlights the importance of pain management not just in the relief of suffering, but also as a preventive activity. Neuroimaging of pain has evolved from providing evidence that pain is processed in the brain at all to a sophisticated, mechanism-orientated research tool that can address a plethora of specific aspects related to the processing, perception, and modulation of pain. Functional brain imaging has provided objective proof of pain perception both in experimentally induced and in disease-related pain. From this, we now know that chronic pain patients display an altered brain activation in response to acute pain stimuli.

There is also some evidence to suggest that brain changes associated with chronic pain may be reversible after effective treatment. In healthy individuals, neuroimaging studies have found that grey matter plasticity can be induced by repetitive experimental noxious stimuli as early as 8 days (after daily pain stimulus for 8 consecutive days), and that this receded between

22 days and 12 months later. That these anatomical changes within the brain occur in the early stages of pain (before pain is labelled as chronic) further suggests that early diagnosis and treatment will be important in preventing chronicity, though this remains to be tested clinically unknown to date.

It is uncertain whether there is pre-existing brain vulnerability to chronic pain, or whether these changes arise as a result of chronic pain. Even if brain responses are found to be tracking pain, these could conceivably represent co-located non-nociceptive functions. Mindful of these caveats, future neuroimaging has the potential to optimize treatment or even offer personalized, improved pain diagnostics in those who cannot communicate this and indicate targets for drug development.

Anxiety, depression, and beliefs about pain in general, are associated with chronic pain and with a poor prognosis in people with various pain conditions. The temporal relationship between chronic pain and mental health remains unclear and is likely bi-directional. There is evidence that top-down (central and cognitive) influences on pain perception may be greater than peripheral input, as exemplified by the analgesic effect of a placebo. It is postulated that placebo analgesia can be potentiated by increasing endogenous opioid tone (e.g. after exercise) and, conversely, that anxiety reduces this endogenous effect. Functional imaging experiments suggest that reducing anxiety can be potentially sustained for a period of up to 3 weeks, with a long-term cognitive shift in nociceptive processing. This suggests an important role for relatively straightforward psychologically based interventions in primary care, aimed at creating and managing expectations, and harnessing the placebo effect.

Further research on the nature and activation of the placebo effect is required to maximize this potential. In depressed patients, neuroimaging has provided evidence of disturbed prefrontal brain activity and a dysfunction of emotion regulation during experimental pain stimulation. This reinforces how factors, such as depression and anxiety associated with chronic pain, become part of the overall condition itself and augment the pain experience. A recent study from the UK in a chronic pain cohort found that sleep problems make depression worse in chronic pain, thus exacerbating a known risk factor.

Chronic pain is more common among those individuals with other chronic diseases than those without and this co-morbidity is associated with significantly poorer self-rated health, lower functional status, and lower ratings of overall quality of care. A recent study using a large New Zealand population cohort, found that the accumulation of stressful life events or physical and mental co-morbidity was independently associated with chronic pain. From an epidemiological point of view, this information suggests that when investigating the contribution of co-morbidity (or adjusting for a confounding effect of co-morbidity), one may need to take into account the presence of specific conditions and the accumulated load (count) of other co-morbidities. Clinically, the implication is that we need to address chronic pain as an important health component of chronic stress, and that doing so successfully might result in a corresponding improvement in overall health.

Recent evidence has also shown that those patients with severe chronic pain have increased risk of mortality, independent of socio-demographic factors. In particular, those individuals reporting severe chronic pain were more than twice as likely to have died 10 years later from heart or lung disease than those reporting no or mild chronic pain. Therefore, one must realize that chronic pain is a serious condition and risk indicator requiring intensive management to minimize the detrimental impact on life and health.

Evidence from birth-cohort studies suggests that chronic pain conditions 'run in families', so that children of parents with chronic pain conditions are more likely to develop pain conditions themselves. Previous work has shown that sensitivity to painful stimuli and pain tolerability are, to a significant extent, determined by one's genetic makeup. More recently, it has been shown that genetic effects in chronic pain are important alongside measured environmental factors in the development and severity of chronic pain. It is unlikely that there is a unique pain gene, rather that multiple genes are associated with the development, processing and perception of chronic pain. The most studied gene in relation to pain is catechol-O-methyltransferase (COMT), an enzyme that degrades neurotransmitters including dopamine.

Many clinical trials have more than one measured outcome variable and several demographic variables of interest. Thus, a number of statistical comparisons will need to be made to analyze and interpret all of the data. The issue of multiple comparisons arises when enough significance tests are done, which leads to the increased likelihood that a test will be statistically significant based on chance alone. Multiple comparisons include repeated analyses of the same outcome variable and comparisons of multiple variables, including testing for differences in baseline characteristics and subgroup analyses. The significance level is also known as the type I error rate and is the probability of a false positive. It is denoted by the Greek letter α. The implication of multiple comparisons is that the investigator should be cautious when interpreting the results.

One way to counter the problem is to require a lower significance level; however, this will reduce the power of the trial. Another alternative is to increase the sample size so that a smaller significance level can be used while maintaining the power of the trial. This option may prove to be quite difficult for most investigators. Many adjustments can be used to approximate or control the significance level that should be used for interpretation of significant findings, including the Bonferroni correction, Holm procedure, and Hochberg procedure. In the case of this investigator who is running 100 separate comparisons with a significance level of 0.05, 5 of them will be significant based on chance alone.

Randomized control trials are comparative studies with an intervention group and a control group, in which the assignment of a subject to a group is determined by a formal process of randomization. In the simplest of terms, randomization is a procedure in which all participants are equally likely to be assigned to either the intervention group or the control group. Randomization is an important concept and is advantageous for many reasons. First, randomization tends to produce comparable groups. This means that measured and unmeasured or unknown characteristics and prognostic factors of the participants will be, on average, evenly balanced between the intervention and control groups. Second, randomization removes the possibility of bias in the allocation of participants to the intervention group or to the control group, also known as selection bias.

Selection bias can be conscious or subconscious and can easily invalidate comparisons, which is why randomization is so important. Finally, randomization provides a sound foundation for valid statistical inference and guarantees the validity of inferential tests of statistical significance. Thus, it ensures independence between assigned treatment and outcome and allows the researcher to state that observed differences between treatment groups are not attributable to chance. Many different procedures can be employed to provide randomization for research studies, including blocked, stratified, adaptive, and play the winner. Based on the 2005 IMMPACT consensus publication, the group recommends use of either the Multidimensional Pain Inventory or the Brief Pain Inventory (BPI) for physical functioning measures. The BPI contains a Pain Interference Scale that provides reliable and valid measures of the interference of pain with physical functioning. The SF-36 Health Survey may be used as a more generic measure of health-related quality of life per IMMPACT's guidelines.

Confidence intervals (CIs) provide a range of plausible values for a population parameter based on the study data results and give an indication of the precision of the measured treatment. The 95% CI is usually reported in the medical literature and represents the range in which there is 95% certainty that the true population parameter will lie. The width of a CI indicates the precision of the estimated parameter in that the wider the CI, the less the precision and higher amount of random error in the measurements.

IMMPACT was formed with the mission to develop consensus reviews and recommendations for improving the design, execution, and interpretation of clinical trials for treatments of pain. IMMPACT recommendations and guidelines have been widely cited and have helped guide chronic pain clinical trial design. Specific areas in which it has made recommendations include core outcome domains, core outcome measures, development of outcome measures, interpretation of clinical importance of treatment outcomes, core outcome and treatment measures for pediatric pain, clinical importance of group differences, analyzing multiple endpoints, research design for confirmatory clinical trials, research design for proof-of-concept studies, and design implications for chronic pain prevention studies. It has been recommended that each of the six core outcome domains should be considered in all clinical trial designs for both efficacy and effectiveness of treatments for chronic pain. Furthermore, if one or more of the domains are not used as an outcome in a study, the reasons for excluding the outcome should be justified a priori.

The six core outcome domains as recommended by IMMPACT are pain, physical functioning, emotional functioning, participant ratings of global improvement and satisfaction with treatment, symptoms and adverse events, and participant disposition. Additional or supplemental outcome domains that researchers may elect to use include role functioning, interpersonal functioning, pharmacoeconomic measures and health care utilization, biological markers, coping, clinician ratings of global improvement, neuropsychological assessments of cognitive and motor function, and suffering or other end-of-life issues. Parametric and nonparametric are two broad classifications of statistical testing procedures. Parametric tests are based on assumptions about the distribution of the underlying population from which the sample was taken. The most common assumption is that the data are normally distributed, also known as a Gaussian distribution.

Characteristics of normal distributions include the following: data are symmetric about the mean, have bell-shaped density curves with a single peak, and are defined by mean (μ) and standard deviation (σ); and mean, median, and mode are the same. In normal distributions, 68% of the total area under the curve is within one standard deviation of the mean, 95% of the total area under the curve is within two standard deviations of the mean, and 99.7% of the total area under the curve is within three standard deviations of the mean. Other factors that determine whether or not a parametric test is suitable include the type of data being analyzed, homogeneity of variances, and whether or not the samples are independent. In contrast, nonparametric statistical procedures rely on few or no assumptions about the shape or parameters of the population distribution from which the sample was taken. It is important to understand when to use a parametric versus a nonparametric statistical procedure. Nonparametric tests use less information and therefore are more conservative tests compared to their parametric alternatives. Thus, if a nonparametric test is used when one has parametric data, the power of the analysis can be decreased, meaning that an individual is less likely to get a significant result when there truly is a significant result.

However, if a parametric test is used wrongly when the data are actually nonparametric, the likelihood of incorrect conclusions increases. In addition to less power, results of nonparametric procedures are more difficult to interpret because many of the tests use rankings of the values in the data rather than using the actual data, which reduces the clinical understanding of the data and results. In a double-blinded study, both patients and providers are unaware of the patients' group assignment. In a triple-blinded study, another group, such as support staff or data analyzers, is also blinded. Randomization is a process of selecting from a group in a manner that makes equal distribution of confounders likely. Randomization will not work as well with small groups. Stratification is a strategy in which patients are intentionally divided by an important characteristic prior to randomization. Confounding occurs when study results are influenced by a factor other than that which is being studied. When a sample is skewed, it may be due to sampling error or related bias. For example, if diabetic patients are more likely than nondiabetics to volunteer for a study, that is a form of volunteer bias. Prior to beginning the study, the investigator determines a priori what are the maximum chances he or she will accept in making type I or type II errors.

The probability of committing a type I error is also known as α or the significance level. A type I error occurs when the null hypothesis is rejected when in reality there actually is no association between the predictor and outcome variable (a false-positive finding). The probability of a type II error is known as β. A type II error occurs when there is a failure to reject the null hypothesis when in reality an association does exist between predictor and outcome (a false-negative finding). Power is specified as $1 - \beta$ and is the probability of correctly rejecting the null hypothesis in the study sample if the actual effect in the population is greater than or equal to the effect size. The crossover design is a special type of a randomized controlled trial (RCT) in which each study treatment is administered at different times to every subject enrolled in the study. Participants in this type of design "crossover" or "switch" from one treatment to another by this strategy, with the intent to estimate differences between them. Typically, half of the participants are randomly assigned to start with one treatment (or control) and then switch to the other treatment (or control). In the case presented in this question, half would start with drug A and switch to drug B, and the other half would start with drug

B and switch to drug A. This is the simplest type of crossover trial and is called the two-treatment, two-period design.

More complex crossover trial designs may be employed in various clinical circumstances. The crossover design has multiple advantages for researchers. One advantage is that it minimizes variability because each participant serves as his or her own control and the subsequent paired analyses substantially increase the statistical power of the trial in that fewer participants are required. Thus, the crossover design takes advantage of making treatment comparisons based on within- rather than between-subject differences. This allows the treatment difference to be estimated with greater precision and less possibility for confounding. Recruitment may also be easier with this type of design because all subjects will receive all treatments under investigation, which may be an attractive attribute for some patients who are concerned about participating in clinical trials in which they may be randomized to a no-treatment or placebo arm.

Some disadvantages of the crossover design are related to the issue of carryover effects and dropouts. Carryover effects are the residual influence of the intervention on the outcome during the period after which it has been discontinued. To reduce carryover effect, the investigator can use an untreated "washout" period between treatments with the hope that the outcome variable will return to its baseline before starting the next intervention. Another concern for carryover effects is if they lead to a permanent change or cure in the underlying condition of the patient. In this instance, the treatment during the second period could appear falsely or artificially superior. Finally, the patients' condition could change in the second treatment phase of the study, which possibly may affect how they respond to the second treatment.

The issue of dropouts is of concern for two reasons. First, the participant is exposed to more drugs or treatments in a crossover trial, increasing the chance of side effects that could contribute to dropping out. Second, the study is usually longer than a regular RCT, thus providing a longer period of opportunity to drop out. The consequences of dropouts are more impactful in a crossover design because the data loss is more significant; for example, if a participant drops out in the second treatment phase, the participant's data cannot be analyzed using only the first phase because that participant was acting as his or her own control and determining a treatment effect cannot occur. NNT (number needed to treat) represents how many people need to be treated or exposed to an intervention in order for one person to have an improved outcome. To calculate NNT, ARR must first be determined. ARR is defined as the difference between the control event rate and the experimental event rate. NNT is equal to the inverse of ARR. Specificity correlates to the proportion of negatives that are correctly identified as such.

Sensitivity is a measure of how likely a test will correctly identify a condition when it is present. Sensitivity is calculated as the number of true positives divided by the sum of true positives and false negatives. Specificity, on the other hand, is a measure of the likelihood that a person without a disease will have a negative test. It is calculated as the number of true negatives divided by the sum of the true negatives and false positives. A positive predictive value is calculated as the number of true positives divided by the sum of true positives and false positives. It is the probability that a patient with a positive test actually has the disease. The negative predictive value, on the other hand, is the number of true negatives divided by the sum of the true negatives and false negatives. Power quantifies the likelihood of identifying a significant effect when it exists. It can be calculated as $1 - \beta$.

References

1. Swain, M.S., Henschke, N., Kamper, S.J., Gobina, I., Ottová-Jordan, V., and Maher, C.G. An international survey of pain in adolescents. BMC Public Health. 2014; 14: 447

2. . Manchikanti, L., Singh, V., Datta, S., Cohen, S.P., and Hirsch, J.A. Comprehensive review of epidemiology, scope, and impact of spinal pain. Pain Physician. 2009; 12: E35–E70

3. INFLAMMATORY PAIN

In order to understand the diagnosis and treatment of painful disorders one must understand the pathologic, and therapeutic differences between inflammatory, neuropathic and nociceptive pain disorders. Inflammation is initiated upon tissue injury and sets off a cascade of biochemical reactions that prime the nervous system for pain sensing. Moreover, long-term inflammation reinforces adaptive changes in the nervous system that can cause the sensation of pain to become exaggerated or inappropriate. For example, inflamed tissue (e.g., an arthritic knee) may be excessively tender and even a light touch might cause pain, a phenomenon known as allodynia. Nociceptive pain does not occur spontaneously, and it must be triggered within the nervous system. This task is accomplished by specialized receptors called nociceptors.

When a person experiences an injury, several inflammatory mediators including prostaglandins, tumor necrosis factor-alpha (TNF-α), Interleukin 1β (IL-1β), and interleukin-6 (IL-6) which are released at the site of the injury and interact with nociceptors, facilitating the transmission of pain signals through the nervous system. If you have a chronic inflammatory condition (e.g., osteoarthritis), then increased levels of inflammatory mediators at the affected site (e.g., a joint), as well as systemically, predispose one to increased pain sensations. Therefore, taking steps to ease inflammation is an effective means of interfering with the process of pain sensitization. This is why drugs like ibuprofen, relieve pain. Unfortunately, though these drugs and others like them are very effective for reducing inflammation and pain, but they can often cause alarming side effects, which compromises their long-term risk vs. benefit profile.

Synovitis is inflammation of the synovium, which is the lining tissue of the joint. It is the clinical hallmark of rheumatoid arthritis) RA and produces pain, swelling, and tenderness of the joint. Other signs of inflammation (e.g., heat and redness) occur less prominently in RA than in other forms of arthritis, such as crystal-induced disease. The diagnosis of RA is supported by the presence of a rheumatoid factor that is an immunoglobulin M (IgM) anti immunoglobulin G (anti-Ig G) antibody. Note, however, that only about 80% of patients with RA display a rheumatoid factor, and that rheumatoid factor can also occur in other clinical settings. The presence of nodules and characteristic deformities (e.g., ulnar deviation, swan neck, and boutonniere deformities of the hands and fingers) substantiate the diagnosis, although these findings indicate more advanced disease and are not invariable. RA is inflammatory, and it initially involves the synovium and secondarily involves the cartilage. In contrast, osteo arthritis (OA) primarily affects the cartilage, with this structure losing its mechanical properties from degeneration or degradation.

Although cartilage in OA lacks the usual signs of inflammation such as an inflammatory cell infiltrate, chondrocytes in the cartilage may produce inflammatory mediators such as interleukin-1 (IL-1) and nitric oxide that cause breakdown of the cartilage matrix. bone. In OA, hypertrophic changes cause bony enlargements called spurs or osteophytes. Inflammation in RA lacks a bony reaction. Heberden and Bouchard's nodes are osteoarthritic bony enlargements in the hands. formation. Spurs or osteophytes represent bony outgrowths around the joint.

OA and RA can be distinguished radiographically because RA causes symmetric joint space narrowing and lacks hypertrophic changes. Note that pain in arthritis can be referred; thus, a painful joint may show only limited change, necessitating radiographic study of a nearby joint to establish the cause. Knee pain, for example, may be referred from the hip. Also Affected by OA include the distal interphalangeal joints of the hands. The lumbar spine is affected by RA as are the metacarpophalangeal joints of hands, wrists, elbows, shoulder, ankles, and the small joints of the feet. DMARDs include methotrexate, leflunomide, tumor necrosis factor (TNF) blockers (etanercept and infliximab), IL-1 receptor antagonist (anakinra), gold salts, penicillamine, hydroxychloroquine, and azathioprine.

More potent immunosuppressants such as cyclosporine and cyclophosphamide are rarely used in RA. Aspirin was the first NSAID developed. It blocks both COX1 and COX2 enzymes. In contrast to nonselective NSAIDs and coxibs, aspirin irreversibly inactivates these enzymes by acetylation. As a result, the actions of aspirin can be long lasting, particularly for the platelets. Samter's syndrome is marked clinically by asthma, nasal polyps, and sensitivity to salicylates. Coxibs do not affect platelet function because they do not inhibit COX1; therefore, they lack benefits in the prevention of cardiovascular or cerebrovascular disease. For patients at risk for these vascular events, a low dose of aspirin can be added to a coxib, although the effect on the GI tract is uncertain. Thus, in the patient with arthritis and a risk for heart disease, aspirin may be used in combination with a coxib. Methotrexate is an antifolate and antimetabolite originally developed to treat malignancy.

In the setting of RA, it is given at much lower doses than when given as an anticancer agent. IL-1 is a proinflammatory cytokine that plays an important role in RA inflammation and damage. Its production is stimulated in part by TNF-α. Among molecules downregulating the action of IL-1, the IL-1 receptor antagonist (IL-1Ra) binds to the receptor for IL-1 and prevents its activation by IL-1. Anakinra (IL-1Ra) is a biological agent that has been approved for the treatment of RA. It is given by subcutaneous administration, although significant doses are required because it must compete with naturally produced IL-1 for effectiveness.

Corticosteroids have potent anti-inflammatory and immunosuppressive actions by which they effectively reduce joint pain and swelling in RA. They interfere with the inflammatory process at various steps. An important action appears to be blockade of the release of arachidonic acid from the cell membrane, limiting substrate for both the lipoxygenase and cyclooxygenase pathways and reducing leukotrienes as well as prostaglandins. Among the indicators of pain that require surgery are pain that lasts all day, pain that awakens the patient from sleep, and pain that requires frequent or continuous narcotics. Disseminated idiopathic skeletal hyperostosis (DISH) is an exaggerated form of osteoarthritis characterized by prominent spine involvement in association with exuberant spur formation. The spine shows calcification of the anterior longitudinal ligament that appears to flow from one vertebra to another in a pattern called "toothpaste" calcification. In this condition, the disc spaces are preserved. Although DISH is commonly associated with back pain, it can also be an incidental finding of chest x-ray.

Polymyalgia rheumatica (PMR) is a painful condition that is frequently acute in onset and causes pain in the shoulder and limb girdles in the absence of other signs of arthritis. It occurs in older individuals (>50 years), shows signs of inflammation with an elevated sedimentation rate (>50 mm/hr.), and responds dramatically to low-dose corticosteroids. Because RA and systemic lupus erythematosus (SLE) can present with a similar pattern, these conditions. Note that pain in arthritis can be referred; thus, a painful joint may show only limited change, necessitating radiographic study of a nearby joint to establish the cause. Knee pain, for example, may be referred from the hip. Also affected by OA include the distal interphalangeal joints of the hands. The lumbar spine is affected by RA as are the metacarpophalangeal joints of hands, wrists, elbows, shoulder, ankles, and the small joints of the feet.

Various foods and dietary patterns are effective in reducing the underlying inflammatory processes associated with chronic disease. A diet high in fruits and vegetables may be one of the best defenses against chronic inflammation. Fruits and vegetables are a highly bioavailable source of vitamins, minerals, fiber, and polyphenols with anti-inflammatory activity. A cross-sectional study investigating self-reported fruit and vegetable intake among adults found that individuals reporting the highest consumption (more than two servings of fruit and three servings of vegetables daily) had significantly lower plasma levels of pro-inflammatory CRP, IL-6, and TNF-alpha as well as decreased biomarkers of oxidative stress. Four to five servings daily each of fruits and vegetables are recommended to combat inflammation and chronic disease.

The Mediterranean diet is characterized by the generous consumption of vegetables, fruits, grains, legumes, and nuts; a minimal intake of red meat and whole-fat dairy products; increased fish consumption; moderate red wine intake; and liberal use of olive oil in cooking and food preparation. Compared with Western diets, the Mediterranean diet is rich in fiber, polyphenols, antioxidants, and omega-3 fatty acids and low in saturated fat and refined carbohydrate. Data from epidemiologic and clinical studies have demonstrated that consuming a Mediterranean-type diet reduces plasma levels of proinflammatory biomarkers, including endothelial adhesion molecules, CRP, TNF-alpha, and NF-kB.

High-fiber, low-GI foods appear to have a beneficial effect on inflammatory biomarkers. Adhering to a low-GI diet for one year resulted in significantly lower plasma levels of CRP in a clinical randomized trial of subjects with type 2 diabetes compared with adhering to high-GI and low-carbohydrate diets. The low-GI diet consisted of high-fiber breakfast cereals, whole grains, and legumes, and provided 52% carbohydrate, an average GI of 55, and 36 g of fiber per day. In contrast, the high-GI diet containing refined cereals, white bread, and potatoes supplied 47% carbohydrate, an average GI of 63, and 21 g of fiber per day; and the low-carbohydrate diet containing nuts, avocados, and olives, provided 39% carbohydrate, an average GI of 59, and 23 g of fiber per day. Whole grain foods consist of the unaltered grain with intact bran and germ components, which are valuable sources of fiber, phytochemicals, vitamins, and minerals. Prospective and clinical studies have suggested that consuming whole grain foods such as oats, barley, and brown rice may help decrease inflammation associated with metabolic syndrome, diabetes, and cardiovascular disease.

Weight loss is known to have beneficial effects on the metabolic syndrome, type 2 diabetes, and other chronic conditions. A small clinical study found that obese individuals who lost 10% or more of their body weight on a low-calorie liquid diet regimen significantly had reduced plasma levels of pro-inflammatory macrophage proteins and pro-inflammatory cytokines IL-6, -15, and -18. The greatest reductions were seen among subjects achieving a weight loss of 14% or more, suggesting that decreased caloric consumption has a beneficial effect on inflammation independent of nutrient intake.

References

1. Estruch R. Anti-inflammatory effects of the Mediterranean diet: the experience of the PREDIMED study. Proc Nutr Soc. 2010;69(3):333-340.

2. Lee HT, Xu H, Nasr SH, Schnermann J, Emala CW (2004) A_1 adenosine receptor knockout mice exhibit increased renal injury following ischemia and reperfusion. Am J Physiol Renal Physiol 286: F298–F306.

4. DIET AND PAIN

The average American consumes approximately 37.8 lb (17.1 kg) of high-fructose corn syrup in 2008, versus 46.7 lb. (21.2 kg) of sucrose. In recent years it has been hypothesized that the increase of high-fructose corn syrup usage in processed foods may be linked to various health conditions, including metabolic syndrome, hypertension, dyslipidemia, hepatic steatosis, insulin resistance, and obesity. However, there is to date little evidence that high-fructose corn syrup is any unhealthier, calorie for calorie, than sucrose or other simple sugars. The fructose content and the fructose-glucose ratio of high-fructose corn syrup do not differ markedly from clarified apple juice.

Some researchers hypothesize that fructose may trigger the process by which fats are formed, to a greater extent than other simple sugars. However, most commonly used blends of high-fructose corn syrup contain a nearly one-to-one ratio of fructose and glucose, just like common sucrose, and should therefore be metabolically identical after the first steps of sucrose metabolism, in which the sucrose is split into fructose and glucose components. At the very least, the increasing prevalence of high-fructose corn syrup has certainly led to an increase in added sugar calories in food, which may reasonably increase the incidence of these and other diseases.

Historically, the extraction of sugar cane juice from the sugarcane plant, and the subsequent domestication of the plant in tropical Southeast Asia sometime around 8,000 B.C. The invention of the manufacture of cane sugar granules from sugarcane juice occurred in India a little over two thousand years ago, followed by improvements in refining the crystal granules in India in the early centuries A.D. Furthermore, the spread of cultivation and manufacture of cane sugar to the medieval Islamic world occurred together with some improvements of the production methods. Subsequently, the spread of the cultivation and manufacture of cane sugar to the West Indies and tropical parts of the Americas began in the 16th century, followed by more intensive improvements in production in the 17th through 19th centuries in that part of the world. The development of beet sugar, high fructose corn syrup and other sweeteners began in the 19th and 20th centuries.

Papuans and Austronesians originally primarily used sugarcane as food for domesticated pigs.   In recent years it has been hypothesized that the increase of high-fructose corn syrup usage in processed foods may be linked to various health conditions, including the metabolic
syndrome, hypertension, dyslipidemia, hepatic steatosis, insulin resistance, and obesity. However, there is to date little evidence that high-fructose corn syrup is any unhealthier, calorie for calorie, than sucrose or other simple sugars. The fructose

content and fructose: glucose ratio of high-fructose corn syrup does not differ markedly from clarified apple juice. Some researchers hypothesize that fructose may trigger the process by which fats are formed, to a greater extent than other simple sugars. However, most commonly used blends of high-fructose corn syrup contain a nearly one-to-one ratio of fructose and glucose, just like common sucrose, and should therefore be metabolically identical after the first steps of sucrose metabolism, in which the sucrose is split into fructose and glucose components. At the very least, the increasing prevalence of high-fructose corn syrup has certainly led to an increase in added sugar calories in food, which may reasonably increase the incidence of these and other diseases including chronic pain.

Americans eat a significant quantity of sugar. According to the U.S. Department of Agriculture (USDA), the average American consumes roughly 47 pounds of cane sugar and 35 pounds of high-fructose corn syrup per year. Sugar is the main ingredient in candy, ice cream and other desserts, but there are also hidden sugars in most processed foods. This includes whole grain breakfast cereals, granola bars, pasta sauce, yogurt, and sports drinks. Research shows that the consumption of foods high in sugar can cause inflammation. Studies measuring inflammation with the blood test C-reactive protein (CRP) discovered that foods with a high concentration of sugar increase CRP levels. This occurs because sugary foods cause a spike in insulin which starts a cascade of biochemical reactions that lead to the production of inflammation. Insulin is secreted from the pancreas and is responsible for taking sugar out of the blood stream and storing it in the cells, which also contributes to the accumulation of fat.

Visceral fat, or stomach fat, itself secretes inflammatory proteins and hormones which generates chronic inflammation. Most forms of joint pain and muscle aches involve inflammation and, even if pain is the result of trauma, symptoms may be exacerbated and prolonged by eating foods high in sugar.   There are lists of "banned" foods deemed sugary: soft drinks, fruit juice, dried fruit, potatoes (the starch eventually converts into glucose), corn, bananas, rice, pasta, honey, and sweets of any kind. Research shows that diet should be an integral part of a pain management program. Getting regular exercise, controlling stress and eating healthy foods all work together to reduce inflammation and chronic pain. The resulting inflammation not only causes pain in the body, but research also shows that an anti-inflammatory diet can ease the pain of fibromyalgia. Sugar also contributes to joint pain and stiffness experienced with aging through a process called glycation.

Glycation occurs when sugar bonds with proteins to form compounds called advanced glycation end products, or AGEs.

These compounds damage cells in the body by speeding up the oxidative process and changing normal cell behavior. AGEs are thought to be a major factor in aging as well as contributing to many age-related chronic diseases. Studies have shown that accumulation of AGEs in joint tissues causes changes in articular cartilage, making the cartilage more susceptible to damage and development of osteoarthritis. Animal studies have shown that sugar can suppress the immune system as yeast and bacteria feed off of it. Sugar also causes an acceleration of aging. Sugar can furthermore attach to proteins and slowly deteriorate the elasticity found in body tissue. This can lead to faster aging in the arteries and organs.

Sugar also increases stress. Sugar can mimic the stress response by raising blood sugar levels, which in turn promotes the body to pump out adrenaline and epinephrine for what the body thinks is much needed energy. These hormones are beneficial, but they can also make you feel more irritable and anxious. The strongest scientific evidence suggests foods rich in a group of antioxidants known as polyphenols can have an anti-inflammatory effect that helps soothe and prevent painful flare-ups. These foods include many of the staples of the Mediterranean diet, such as whole fruits (especially all types of berries), dark green leafy vegetables, nuts, legumes, and whole grains. Some research has suggested that omega-3 fatty acids, which are found in olive oil, flaxseed oil, and fatty fish (like salmon, sardines, and mackerel), also may help control inflammation.

References

1. Campbell-McBride N. Gut and Psychology Syndrome. [Cambridge, U.K.: Medinform Pub.]; 2010.

2. 2.Carlsen M, Halvorsen B, Holte K et al. The total antioxidant content of more than 3100 foods, beverages, spices, herbs and supplements used worldwide. Nutrition Journal. 2010;9(1):3. doi:10.1186/1475-2891-9-3.

3. DeGroot J, Verzijl N, Jacobs KM, et al. Accumulation of advanced glycation end products reduces chondrocyte-mediated extracellular matrix turnover in human articular cartilage. Osteoarthritis Cartilage. 2001;9(8):720–6.

4. Dirsch V, Vollmar A. Ajoene, a natural product with non-steroidal anti-inflammatory drug (NSAID)-like properties? Biochemical Pharmacology. 2001;61(5):587-593. doi:10.1016/s0006-2952(00)00580-3.

5. PAIN NEUROPHYSIOLOGY

When a patient has severe pain complaints and seeks treatment, it is hard to sort out the myths from the realities. To feel less pain, does one rest in bed or go walking? Should an individual talk to a specialist about taking potent drugs or should the patient refrain from this behavior? Chronic pain can be a serious and incapacitating medical condition. Many people suffering with chronic pain are so desperate for help that they're willing to believe whatever advertising babble they are exposed to, and as a result buy into some chronic pain fables that could be risky, expensive and even dangerous. Treating chronic pain is not simple. Remedying the cause of one's pain does resolve the pain in many instances but not always. Anyone with chronic pain must see a pain physician to comprehend if there's a correctable or a non-correctable disease which causes chronic pain. For example, if a patient has acute pain related to an appendicitis, surgery should correct the problem. If a patient on the other hand, has rheumatoid arthritis, the patient will have chronic pain as this a permanent disease entity.

In many cases, the relationship of an underlying cause of one's pain perception is more complicated. Painful diseases might be chronic and hard to control. Sometimes pain lingers even after the original cause seems to have been resolved. People with chronic pain often need a double approach: 1. get care for the underlying cause and 2. independently treat the pain itself. That often means seeing a pain management specialist as well as other doctors. Over time, chronic pain if not treated can lead to sleep deprivation, social isolation, depression and other problems. There's an immense consequence to treatment with opioids as well. Opioids are not effective with all types of pain. They can, furthermore, cause unpleasant side effects. A physical dependency can develop if pain management and treatment is not monitored. This is not an addiction, but some bodies adapt to the medication. Over time they need higher doses to get the same level of relief.

Opioid drugs can, furthermore, increase the risk that other treatment approaches will fail and there is substantiation that opioids can result in chronic pain in some patients. For example, a person with mild, occasional headaches might develop chronic, debilitating ones after using high doses of opioids for a certain amount of time. There is not a universal "unsurpassed" treatment for chronic pain. It is just another tool among many others, from anti-inflammatory medicines to alternative therapies such as acupuncture.

Some patients with chronic pain often have a misunderstanding that they believe that they will be able to find the one perfect treatment that will remedy their pain. This perfect remedy does not exist. The purpose of this book is to explain the different types of pain and what can be done to decrease this pain. It may be a new drug or a new surgical technique that they read about in the paper or saw an advertisement on an infomercial. They then rapidly anticipate that there's one solution for them that will take their pain away entirely. Even with good medical treatment, chronic pain may never go away. It's unfortunate but true. Someone who has had ongoing back pain for 15 years shouldn't expect that after few visits to a pain doctor that they will be cured. Managing chronic pain is usually a long process. Even if physicians cannot make the chronic pain disappear completely, treatment can nevertheless make a pronounced difference in many patients. The most important concept is how the pain affects a patient's quality of life.

A patient may continue to have some pain after treatment but if the pain management restores a patient's ability to do tasks that the chronic pain prevented, it is then meaningful and worthwhile. Patients should be aware that chronic pain can provide medical specialists a significant income by addicting patients with potent opioids and by doing multiple injections that provide patients at most only temporary pain relief. The purpose of this book is to present the reader with a comprehensive description of the various categories of pain syndromes and what modalities can attenuate these various pain syndromes and to alert individuals that proper nutrition and sugar elimination may also decrease one's chronic pain. The information in the first few chapters of this book may seem redundant, but knowledge of the anatomy and physiology of the different types of pain is imperative to understand so that pain syndromes can be treated in a rational manner. "Granny Smith's tonic" or "Dr. Joe's multiple steroid injections" in other words do not cure all pain syndromes.

In order to understand essential pain concepts, one should be familiar with the basic neurophysiology of the parts of the nervous system involved in pain transmission and interpretation. The nervous system is nature's way of sending instructions from one part of the body to another. Signals that begin in the central nervous system (usually the brain but sometimes the spinal cord) move toward the periphery to locations such as the limbs or internal organs and direct the target to do something. Nerves function by transmitting electrochemical impulses they receive from the brain or other nerves to nerves "downstream" or to the cells, organs or tissues at which these nerves terminate. It is conventional, to describe nerve types on the basis of their function: motor, sensory, autonomic or cranial. Motor neurons send impulses from the brain and spinal cord to the muscles throughout the body. Motor nerve damage can lead to weakness in the muscle or muscles supplied and atrophy of those muscles as well.

The sciatic nerve that runs from the lower back through the buttocks to serve the entire leg is actually a bundle of many different nerves, some of them motor neurons serving the thigh, hamstring, calves and feet. Sensory nerves (sensory neurons) send impulses in the opposite direction from motor neurons.

They collect information about pain, pressure, temperature and so on from sensors in the skin, muscles and internal organs and send it back to the spinal cord and the brain. Sensory nerves are even capable of relaying information about motion (apart from what the eyes themselves do). Sensory nerve damage may cause tingling, numbness, pain and oversensitivity. The autonomic nervous system regulates the activity of heart muscle, smooth muscle like that in the stomach and the lining of other organs, and glands. These nerves control functions not under conscious control.

The autonomic nervous system includes two functional divisions: the sympathetic nervous system, involved in speeding up heart rate and other "fight or flight" responses; and the parasympathetic nervous system, which regulates digestion, excretion and other metabolic activities. A ganglion is a group of neuron cell bodies in the periphery. Ganglia can be categorized, for the most part, as either sensory ganglia or autonomic ganglia, referring to their primary functions. The most common type of sensory ganglion is a dorsal (posterior) root ganglion. These ganglia are the cell bodies of neurons with axons that are sensory endings in the periphery, such as in the skin, and that extend into the CNS through the dorsal nerve root. The ganglion is an enlargement of the nerve root.

The human brain is the central organ of the human nervous

system, and with the spinal cord makes up the central nervous system. The brain consists of the cerebrum, the brainstem, and the cerebellum. It controls most of the activities of the body, processing, integrating, and coordinating the information it receives from the sense organs and making decisions as to the instructions sent to the rest of the body. The brain is contained in, and protected by, the skull bones of the head. The cerebrum is the most significant part of the human brain. It is divided into two cerebral hemispheres. The cerebral cortex is an outer layer of grey matter, covering the core of the white matter. The cortex is split into the neocortex and the much smaller allocortex. The neocortex is made up of six neuronal layers, while the allocortex has three or four. Each hemisphere is conventionally divided into four lobes: the frontal, temporal, parietal, and occipital lobes.

The frontal lobe is associated with executive functions including self-control, planning, reasoning, and abstract thought, while the occipital lobe is dedicated to vision. Within each lobe, cortical areas are associated with specific functions, such as the sensory, motor and association regions. Although the left and right hemispheres are broadly similar in shape and function, some functions are associated with one side, such as language in the left and visual-spatial ability in the right. Commissural nerve tracts connect the hemispheres, the largest being the corpus callosum.

The brainstem connects the cerebrum to the spinal cord. The brainstem consists of the midbrain, the pons, and the medulla oblongata. The cerebellum is connected to the brainstem by pairs of tracts. Within the cerebrum is the ventricular system, consisting of four interconnected ventricles in which cerebrospinal fluid is produced and circulated. Underneath the cerebral cortex are several vital structures, including the thalamus, the epithalamus, the pineal gland, the hypothalamus, the pituitary gland, and the subthalamus; the limbic structures, including the amygdala and the hippocampus; the claustrum, the various nuclei of the basal ganglia; the basal forebrain structures, and the three circumventricular organs. The cells of the brain include neurons and supportive glial cells. There are more than 86 billion neurons in the brain and a more or less equal number of other cells. Brain activity is made possible by the interconnections of neurons and their release of neurotransmitters in response to nerve impulses. Neurons connect to form neural pathways, neural circuits, and elaborate network systems.

The process of neurotransmission drives the whole circuitry. The cerebrum, consisting of the cerebral hemispheres, forms the most significant part of the brain and overlies the other brain structures. The outer region of the hemispheres, the cerebral cortex, is grey matter, consisting of cortical layers of neurons. Each hemisphere is divided into four main lobes: the frontal lobe, parietal lobe, temporal lobe, and occipital lobe. Three other lobes are included by some sources which are a central lobe, a limbic lobe, and an insular lobe. The central lobe comprises the precentral gyrus and the postcentral gyrus and is included since it forms a distinct functional role.   The brainstem, which resembles a stalk, attaches to and leaves the cerebrum at the start of the midbrain area. The brainstem includes the midbrain, the pons, and the medulla oblongata. Behind the brainstem is the cerebellum.

Three membranes called meninges cover the cerebrum, brainstem, cerebellum, and spinal cord. The membranes are the tough dura mater; the middle arachnoid mater and the more delicate inner pia mater. Between the arachnoid mater and the pia mater is the subarachnoid space and subarachnoid cisterns, which contain the cerebrospinal fluid. The outermost membrane of the cerebral cortex is the basement membrane of the pia mater called the glia limitans and is an integral part of the blood-brain barrier. The living brain is very soft, having a gel-like consistency similar to jello. The cortical layers of neurons constitute much of the cerebral grey matter, while the deeper subcortical regions of myelinated axons, make up the white matter. The white matter of the brain makes up about one half of the total brain volume. The cerebrum is the most substantial part of the brain and is divided into left and right hemispheres. Five commissures connect the hemispheres that span the longitudinal fissure, the largest of these is the corpus callosum. Each hemisphere is conventionally divided into four main lobes; the frontal lobe, parietal lobe, temporal lobe, and occipital lobe, named according to the skull bones that overlie them. Each lobe is associated with one or two specialized functions though there is some functional overlap between them. The surface of the brain is folded into ridges (gyri) and grooves (sulci), many of which are named, usually according to their position, such as the frontal gyrus of the frontal lobe or the central sulcus separating the central regions of the hemispheres. There are many small variations in the secondary and tertiary folds.

The cortex of the brain is divided into two main functional areas, a motor and a sensory cortex. The primary motor cortex, which sends axons down to motor neurons in the brainstem and spinal cord, occupies the rear portion of the frontal lobe, directly in front of the somatosensory area. The primary sensory areas receive signals from the sensory nerves and tracts by way of relay nuclei in the thalamus. Primary sensory areas include the visual cortex of the occipital lobe, the auditory cortex in parts of the temporal lobe and insular cortex, and the somatosensory cortex in the parietal lobe. The remaining parts of the cortex are called the association areas. These areas receive input from the sensory areas and lower parts of the brain and are involved in the complex cognitive processes of perception, thought, and decision-making.

The main functions of the frontal lobe are to control attention, abstract thinking, behavior, problem-solving tasks, and physical reactions and personality. The occipital lobe is the smallest lobe; its primary functions are visual reception, visual-spatial processing, movement, and color recognition. There is a smaller occipital lobule in the lobe known as the cuneus. The temporal lobe controls auditory and visual memories, language, and some hearing and speech. The cerebrum contains the ventricles where the cerebrospinal fluid is produced and circulated. Below the corpus callosum is the septum pellucidum, a membrane that separates the lateral ventricles. Beneath the lateral ventricles is the thalamus and to the front and below this is the hypothalamus. The hypothalamus leads on to the pituitary gland.

At the back of the thalamus is the brainstem. The basal ganglia are a set of structures deep within the hemispheres involved in behavior and movement regulation. The most significant component is the striatum, others are the globus pallidus, the substantia niagra, and the subthalamic nucleus. Part of the dorsal striatum, the putamen, and the globus pallidus, lie separated from the lateral ventricles and thalamus by the internal capsule, whereas the caudate nucleus stretches around and abuts the lateral ventricles on their outer sides. At the deepest part of the lateral sulcus between the insular cortex and the striatum is a thin neuronal sheet called the claustrum.

Below and in front of the striatum are many basal forebrain structures. These structures are essential in producing acetylcholine. The brainstem lies beneath the cerebrum and consists of the midbrain, pons, and medulla. It lies in the back part of the skull, resting on the part of the base known as the clivus, and ends at the foramen magnum, a large opening in the occipital bone. The brainstem continues below this as the spinal cord protected by the vertebral column. Ten of the twelve pairs of cranial nerves emerge directly from the brainstem. The brainstem also contains many cranial nerve nuclei and nuclei of peripheral nerves, as well as nuclei involved in the regulation of many essential processes including breathing, control of eye movements and balance.

The reticular formation, a network of nuclei of ill-defined formation, is present within and along the length of the brainstem. Many nerve tracts, which transmit information to and from the cerebral cortex to the rest of the body, pass through the brainstem. The larger arteries throughout the brain supply blood to smaller capillaries. These smallest of blood vessels in the brain, are lined with cells joined by tight junctions, and so fluids do not seep in or leak out to the same degree as they do in other capillaries, thereby creating the blood-brain barrier. From the joints, the brain receives information about the joint position.

The sensory cortex is found just near the motor cortex, and, like the motor cortex, has areas related to sensation from different body parts. Sensation collected by a sensory receptor on the skin is changed to a nerve signal, that is passed up a series of neurons through tracts in the spinal cord. The dorsal column-medial lemniscus pathway contains information about fine touch, vibration, and position of joints. Neurons travel up the back part of the spinal cord to the back part of the medulla, where they connect with second-order neurons that immediately swap sides. These neurons then travel upwards into the ventral basal complex in the thalamus where they connect with third-order neurons and travel up to the sensory cortex.

The spinothalamic tract carries information about pain, temperature, and gross touch. Neurons travel up the spinal cord and connect with second-order neurons in the formation of the brainstem for pain and temperature, and also at the ventro basal complex of the medulla for gross touch. Chemical neurotransmitters include dopamine, serotonin, GABA, glutamate, and acetylcholine. GABA is the major inhibitory neurotransmitter in the brain, and glutamate is the major excitatory neurotransmitter. A neural pathway is a connection formed by axons that project from neurons to make synapses onto neurons in another location, to enable a signal to be sent from one region of the nervous system to another. Neurons are connected by a single axon, or by a bundle of axons known as a nerve tract, or fasciculus. Shorter neural pathways are found within the grey matter in the brain, whereas longer projections, made up of myelinated axons, constitute white matter. In general, neurons receive information either at their dendrites or cell bodies. The axon of a nerve cell is, in general, responsible for transmitting information over a relatively long distance. Therefore, most neural pathways are made up of axons.

If the axons have myelin sheaths, then the pathway appears bright white because myelin is primarily lipid. The spinal cord functions primarily in the transmission of nerve signals from the motor cortex to the body, and from the afferent fibers of the sensory neurons to the sensory cortex. It is also a center for coordinating many reflexes and contains reflex arcs that can independently control reflexes. It is also the location of groups of spinal interneurons that make up the neural circuits known as central pattern generators. These circuits are responsible for controlling motor instructions for rhythmic movements such as walking. The dorsal roots are afferent fascicles, receiving sensory information from the skin, muscles, and visceral organs to be relayed to the brain. The roots terminate in dorsal root ganglia, which are composed of the cell bodies of the corresponding neurons. Ventral roots consist of efferent fibers that arise from motor neurons whose cell bodies are found in the ventral (or anterior) gray horns of the spinal cord. The somatosensory organization is divided into the dorsal column-medial lemniscus tract (the touch/proprioception/vibration sensory pathway) and the anterolateral system, or ALS (the pain/temperature sensory pathway).

Both sensory pathways use three different neurons to get information from sensory receptors at the periphery to the cerebral cortex. These neurons are designated primary, secondary and tertiary sensory neurons. In both pathways, primary sensory neuron cell bodies are found in the dorsal root ganglia, and their central axons project into the spinal cord. The anterolateral system works somewhat differently. Its primary neurons axons enter the spinal cord and then ascend one to two levels before synapsing in the substantia gelatinosa. The tract that ascends before synapsing is known as Lissauer's tract. After synapsing, secondary axons decussate and ascend in the anterior lateral portion of the spinal cord as the spinothalamic tract. This tract ascends to the VPLN, where it synapses on tertiary neurons. Tertiary neuronal axons then travel to the primary sensory cortex via the posterior limb of the internal capsule.

Some of the "pain fibers" in the ALS deviate from their pathway towards the VPLN. In one such deviation, axons travel towards the reticular formation in the midbrain. The reticular formation then projects to several places including the hippocampus (to create memories about the pain), the central median nucleus (to cause diffuse, non-specific pain) and various parts of the cortex. Additionally, some ALS axons project to the periaqueductal gray in the pons, and the axons forming the periaqueductal gray then project to the nucleus raphes magnus, which projects back down to where the pain signal is coming from and inhibits it. This helps control the sensation of pain to some degree.

With respect to nutrition, the aim of a study previously published was to investigate if food could reduce pain perception in a group of 16 healthy human volunteers (8 male and 8 female), and to explore the differential effects of macronutrient composition on the response to cold-induced pain. All subjects underwent the cold pressor test (CPT) on 3 occasions in a counterbalanced order, before and after administration of isoenergetic high-fat low-carbohydrate (CHO) and high-CHO low-fat meals, and when no meal was given. The CPT was carried out four times on each test day, once before the meal, and 0.5, 1.5, and 2.5 h after the meal, and at the equivalent times on the day when no food was given. Radial pulse and blood pressure measurements and visual analogue scales of mood/emotional state were carried out before and after each CPT. Mean pain scores were significantly reduced following both meals compared with the no-food condition. The maximum reduction in pain occurred 1.5 h after ingestion, and a significantly greater effect was exerted by the high-fat low-CHO meal compared with the high-CHO low-fat meal. These results demonstrate that food, particularly when rich in fat, significantly reduces the pain induced by the cold pressor stimulus in healthy human subjects.

Dietary habits are fundamental issues to assess when modulating health and well-being; however, different nutritional panels may help individuals prevent acute and chronic pain. Many substances, known to be active antioxidants and anti-inflammatory compounds, should serve this fundamental task. Antinociceptive and analgesic natural compounds include flavonoids, terumbone from ginger root, curcuminoids, ω-3 polyunsaturated fatty acids, and taurine. Furthermore, correct intake of trace elements and minerals is strategic to reduce inflammation-related pain.

References

1. 2019 Apr 26; 66:153-165. doi: 10.1016/j.nut.2019.04.007. [Epub ahead of print] Has human diet a role in reducing nociception related to inflammation and chronic pain? Bjørklund G1, Aaseth J2, Doşa MD3, Pivina L4, Dadar M5, Pen JJ6, Chirumbolo S7.

2. 2. Zmarzty SA1, Wells AS, Read NW. Brain anatomy and physiology, Physiol Behav. 1997 Jul;62(1):185-91. The influence of food on pain perception in healthy human volunteers.

6. BRAIN PHYSIOLOGY

Sensation collected by a sensory receptor on the skin is changed to an electrical nerve signal and that current is passed up a series of neurons through tracts in the spinal cord. The dorsal column medial lemniscus pathway contains information about fine touch, vibration and position of joints. Neurons travel up the back part of the spinal cord to the back part of the medulla, where they connect with second order neurons that immediately swap sides. These neurons then travel upwards into the ventro basal complex in the thalamus where they connect with third-order neurons and travel up to the sensory cortex. The spinothalamic tract carries information about pain, temperature, and gross touch. Neurons travel up the spinal cord and connect with second-order neurons in the formation of the brainstem for pain and temperature, and also at the complex of the medulla for gross touch.

Chemical neurotransmitters in a body include the following: serotonin, GABA, glutamate, and acetylcholine. GABA is the major inhibitory neurotransmitter in the brain, and glutamate is the major excitatory neurotransmitter. A neural pathway is the connection formed by axons that project from neurons to make synapses onto neurons in another location, to enable a signal to be sent from one region of the nervous system to another. Neurons are connected by a single axon, or by a bundle of axons known as a nerve tract, or fasciculus. Shorter neural pathways are found within grey matter in the brain, whereas longer projections, made up of myelinated axons, constitue white matter.

In general, neurons receive information either at their dendrites or cell bodies. The axon of a nerve cell is, in general, responsible for transmitting information over a relatively long distance. Therefore, most neural pathways are made up of axons. If the axons have myelin sheaths, then the pathway appears bright white because myelin is primarily lipid. The spinal cord functions primarily in the transmission of nerve signals from the motor cortex to the body, and from the afferent fibers of the sensory neurons to the sensory cortex. It is also a center for coordinating many reflexes and contains reflex arcs that can independently control reflexes. It is also the location of groups of spinal interneurons that make up the neural circuits known as central pattern generators.

These circuits are responsible for controlling motor instructions for rhythmic movements such as walking. The dorsal roots are afferent fascicles, receiving sensory information from the skin, muscles, and visceral organs to be relayed to the brain. The roots terminate in dorsal root ganglion, which are composed of the cell bodies of the corresponding neurons. Ventral roots consist of efferent fibers that arise from motor neurons whose cell bodies are found in the ventral (or anterior) gray horns of the spinal cord. Somatosensory organization is divided into the dorsal column-medial lemniscus tract (the touch/proprioception/vibration sensory pathway) and the anterolateral system, or ALS (the pain/temperature sensory pathway).

Both sensory pathways use three different neurons to get information from sensory receptors at the periphery to the cerebral cortex. These neurons are designated primary, secondary and tertiary sensory neurons. In both pathways, primary sensory neuron cell bodies are found in the dorsal root ganglion, and their central axons project into the spinal cord. The anterolateral system works somewhat differently. Its primary neurons axons enter the spinal cord and then ascend one to two levels before synapsing in the substantia gelatinosa. The tract that ascends before synapsing is known as Lissauer's tract. After synapsing, secondary axons decussate and ascend in the anterior lateral portion of the spinal cord as the spinothalamic tract. This tract ascends all the way to the VPLN, where it synapses on tertiary neurons.

Tertiary neuronal axons then travel to the primary sensory cortex via the posterior limb of the internal capsule. Some of the "pain fibers" in the ALS deviate from their pathway towards the VPLN. In one such deviation, axons travel towards the reticular formation in the midbrain. The reticular formation then projects to a number of places including the hippocampus (to create memories about the pain), the centro median nucleus (to cause diffuse, non-specific pain) and various parts of the cortex. Additionally, some ALS axons project to the peri aqueductal gray matter in the pons, and the axons forming the periaqueductal gray then project to the nucleus raphe magnus, which projects back down to where the pain signal is coming from and inhibits it. This helps control the sensation of pain to some degree.

The modulation of pain by electrical brain stimulation results from the activation of descending inhibitory fibers, which modulate (block) the input and output of laminae I, II, V and VII neurons. The route from the PAG to the spinal cord is not direct. It appears to involve a link with the 5-HT-rich raphe nuclei, as well as norepinephrine (NE) from the locus coeruleus (LC) and dopamine (DA) from the ventral tegmental area (VTA). Axons from the raphe nuclei, locus coeruleus and VTA project to the spinal cord dorsal horn by way of the DLF to terminate in lamina I, II and IV to VII (i.e., stimulation of NRM, VTA and LC inhibits the neuronal activity of lamina I, II and IV to VII neurons). Opioid and serotonergic antagonists reverse both local opiate analgesia and brain-stimulation produced analgesia. This suggests that OA and SPA are produced via the same descending inhibitory system.

The aim of a previous study was to investigate if food could reduce pain perception in a group of 16 healthy human volunteers (8 male and 8 female), and to explore the differential effects of macronutrient composition on the response to cold-induced pain. All subjects underwent the cold pressor test (CPT) on 3 occasions in a counterbalanced order, before and after administration of isoenergetic high-fat low-carbohydrate (CHO) and high-CHO low-fat meals, and when no meal was given. The CPT was carried out 4 times on each test day, once before the meal, and 0.5, 1.5, and 2.5 h after the meal, and at the equivalent times on the day when no food was given. Radial pulse and blood pressure measurements and visual analogue scales of mood/emotional state were carried out before and after each CPT. Mean pain scores were significantly reduced following both meals compared with the no-food condition. The maximum reduction in pain occurred 1.5 h after ingestion, and a significantly greater effect was exerted by the high-fat low-CHO meal compared with the high-CHO low-fat meal. These results demonstrate that food, particularly when rich in fat, significantly reduces the pain induced by the cold pressor stimulus in healthy human subjects. In conclusion, in the CNS, much of the information from the nociceptive afferent fibers results from excitatory discharges of multi receptive neurons.

The pain information in the CNS is controlled by ascending and descending inhibitory systems, using endogenous opioids, or other endogenous substances like serotonin as inhibitory mediators. In addition, a powerful inhibition of pain-related information occurs in the spinal cord. These inhibitory systems can be activated by brain stimulation, intracerebral microinjection of morphine, and peripheral nerve stimulation. Centrally acting analgesic drugs activate these inhibitory control systems. However, pain is a complex perception that is influenced also by prior experience and by the context within which the noxious stimulus occurs. This sensation is also influenced by emotional state. Therefore, the response to pain varies from subject to subject.

References

1. Zmarzty SA1, Wells AS, Read NW. Physiol Behav. 1997 Jul;62(1):185-91. The influence of food on pain perception in healthy human volunteers.

2. Anjana, Yumnam, and Keisam Reetu. "Effect of food intake on pain perception in healthy human subjects." Journal of Evolution of Medical and Dental Sciences, vol. 3, no. 29, 2014, p. 7984+. Gale Academic Onefile, Accessed 25 Sept. 2019.

7. PAIN OVERVIW

The word "pain" is derived from the Latin word poena that means punishment. St. Augustine wrote in the 5th century that all diseases afflicting Christians were derived from demons. Ancient tribal concepts of pain were based on beliefs that evil spirits were sent as punishment from their gods to invade one's body and cause severe pain. In the book of Genesis, Eve was condemned to pain during childbirth as a result of her encounter with the devil in the Garden of Eden. It has been reported that a shaman could suck an evil spirit from a wound to decrease one's pain. The ancient Greeks such as Aristotle were the first individuals who believed that pain was derived from various nerves in the body. The exact cause of pain was unknown to them. Unfortunately, not unlike ancient times, the diagnosis and treatment of many chronic painful conditions today remain mostly guesswork in both young and elderly patients. Pain medicine is, for the most part, subjectively based, because pain is a subjective symptom while other medical specialties are based upon objective curative evidence. Pain in general is not totally bad. Pain is a protective mechanism that warns a patient that the body has something wrong in some location. The International Association for the Study of Pain defines pain as" an unpleasant sensory and emotional experience associated with tissue injury as a result of trauma (e.g. bone fracture) or disease (e.g. cancer, shingles). Pain has psychological effects in some instances especially when pain is severe. Pain may cause anxiety and depression. Acute pain is associated with injury, bone fractures, surgery or sprains and strains. Once these entities have healed, sometimes the pain continues which causes chronic pain (pain lasting over 90 days). Arthritis is an example of chronic pain. Arthritic pain is caused by continuous joint destruction. However, once the pain becomes chronic, the pain becomes a problem.

Not only does pain become a personal problem but pain can become a social problem with creation of family problems, loss of self-esteem, lost wages etc. Fibromyalgia patients have alterations in CNS anatomy, physiology, and chemistry that potentially contribute to the symptoms experienced by these patients. The impact of age and gender on experimental pressure pain detection thresholds and pressure pain tolerance thresholds and participants' self-reports of pain intensity and unpleasantness at supra threshold and sub-threshold levels are varied. The intensity and unpleasantness of the pain stimulus were significantly rated lower in the elderly as compared with the young. No gender differences, however, were observed in the report of intensity and unpleasantness of the stimulations. The elderly appraise pain experiences using different psychological strategies. Pain impulses are, in essence, electrical signals that travel from various areas of the body such as the extremities, heart, appendix, etc. to the spinal cord and eventually reach the brain where the pain signals are processed like data in a computer.

Pain is produced by unpleasant stimuli to nerve endings throughout the body which include chemical, extreme heat cold and mechanical injury. These nerve endings are silent until mechanical, heat or cold trauma injures tissue. In order to experience pain, a patient needs pain a receptor and a nerve fiber that transmits pain to travel from the area of the pain to the spinal cord and then to the brain. As people age, they become more motivated to maximize positive emotions and minimize negative ones. Nerves, which conduct pain impulses to the spinal cord, are composed of neurons (nerve cells) that make up nerve fibers that form neurons. Two common pain fibers are the C fibers and the A-delta fibers. A-delta fibers conduct fast onset sharp pain impulses. The C fibers conduct slow onset dull, aching or burning pain. Other types of fibers that transmit touch and vibration do not cause pain in most instances. However, these fibers can become hypersensitive and may contribute to the total pain experience. A neuron is an electrically excitable cell in the nervous system that processes and transmits information. Neurons are the significant core components of the brain and spinal cord as well as peripheral nerves. Neurons are typically composed of a cell body, a dendrite and an axon. Neurons receive input from dendrites and transmit output via the axon. When noxious stimuli impinge upon the body from external or internal sources, information regarding the damaging impact of these stimuli on bodily tissues is transduced through neural pathways and transmitted through the peripheral nervous system to the central and autonomic nervous systems. This form of information processing is known as nociception.

The perception of pain occurs when stimulation of nociceptors is intense enough to activate Aδ fibers, resulting in a subjective experience of a sharp, prickling pain. As stimulus strength increases, C fibers are recruited, and the individual experiences an intense, burning pain that continues after the cessation of the stimulus. These types of experiences occur during the two phases of pain perception that occur following an acute injury. The first phase, which is not particularly intense, comes immediately after the painful stimulus and is known as fast pain. The second phase, known as slow pain, is more unpleasant, less discretely localized, and occurs after a longer delay. Activation of nociceptors is transduced along the axons of peripheral nerves which terminate in the dorsal horn of the spine. There, messages are relayed up the spinal cord and through the spinothalamic tract to output on the thalamus. In turn, the thalamus serves as the major "relay station" for sensory information to the cerebral cortex. Nociceptive pathways terminate in discrete subdivisions of thalamic nuclei in the brain known as the ventral posterior lateral nucleus and the ventromedial nucleus. From these nuclei, nociceptive information is relayed to various brain cortical and subcortical regions, including the amygdala, hypothalamus, periaqueductal grey, basal ganglia, and regions of cerebral cortex. Most notably, the insula and anterior cingulate cortex are consistently activated when nociceptors are stimulated by noxious stimuli, and activation in these brain regions is associated with the subjective experience of pain. In turn, these integrated thalamocortical and corticolimbic structures, which collectively have been termed the pain "neuromatrix," process somatosensory input and output neural impulses which influence nociception and pain perception. Perception of pain occurs when stimulation of nociceptors is intense enough to activate $A\delta$ fibers, resulting in a subjective experience of a sharp, prickling pain. As the stimulus strength increases, C fibers are recruited, and the individual experiences an intense, burning pain that continues after the cessation of the stimulus. These types of experiences occur during the two phases of pain perception that occur following an acute injury. The first phase, which is not particularly intense, comes immediately after the painful stimulus and is known as fast pain.

The second phase, known as slow pain, is more unpleasant, less discretely localized, and occurs after a longer delay. Activation of nociceptors is transduced along the axons of peripheral nerves which terminate in the dorsal horn of the spine. There, messages are relayed up the spinal cord and through the spinothalamic tract to output on the thalamus. In turn, the thalamus serves as the major "relay station" for sensory information to the cerebral cortex. Nociceptive pathways terminate in discrete subdivisions of thalamic nuclei known as the ventral posterior lateral nucleus and the ventromedial nucleus. From these nuclei, nociceptive information is relayed to various cortical and subcortical regions, including the amygdala, hypothalamus, periaqueductal grey, basal ganglia, and regions of cerebral cortex. Most notably, the insula and anterior cingulate cortex are consistently activated when nociceptors are stimulated by noxious stimuli, and activation in these brain regions is associated with the subjective experience of pain. In turn, these integrated thalamocortical and corticolimbic structures, which collectively have been termed the pain "neuromatrix," process somatosensory input and output neural impulses which influence nociception and pain perception.

Neurons are the building blocks of nerves. In other words, multitudes of neurons are necessary to form a nerve. Nerves that are bundled together exist outside of the central nervous system are called a ganglion. The stellate ganglion in the neck is an example. Various ganglia may form a plexus. An example of a plexus is the celiac plexus. A nerve is composed of neurons. A neuron has one axon that takes nerve signals away from the neuron. The long end of the axon communicates with multiple dendrites. Action potentials generated by the neuron initiate pain signals. If the skin is pinched a mechanical pain receptor begins an action potential. An action potential begins after a depolarization could cause a membrane transitory modification, turning prevalently permeable to sodium ions more than to potassium ions. Sodium permeability can cause an action potential. A neuropathy generates a local accumulation of nerve sodium channels. This model seems to be the basis of neuron hyper excitability. Calcium channels have also an important role in cell function. An intra-cellular calcium increase contributes to a depolarization processes, through kinase and determines the phosphorylation of membrane proteins that can make powerful the efficacy of the channels them-selves.

Following an acute injury, AMPA receptors are stimulated, which cause sharp pain. There are receptors that are present in the spinal cord are called NMDA (N-methyl-D-aspartate) receptors and cause chronic pain. When these NMDA receptors are stimulated, pain becomes more severe and this extreme pain is maintained. The brain is responsible for the suffering associated with severe pain. Pain results in bodily responses, especially with respect to the cardiovascular system (heart rate increases, blood pressure increases, renal arteries constrict, etc.). When the pain is severe, the brain can cause the body to increase both the heart rate and blood pressure. Extreme pain can also result in profuse sweating as well as nausea and vomiting. There are different types of nerve endings throughout the body. The pain nerve endings become hyper excitable when stimulated by injury, inflammation or a tumor. Occasionally, the nerve endings remain irritable even after the painful stimulus has been removed which cause chronic pain. Pain signals from areas in the body reach the brain by four processes (transduction, transmission, modulation and perception). Axons carry pain fibers away from a neuron and direct them to the dendrites of the next neuron until they terminate in the brain or spinal cord. The axons and dendrites do not touch. They form synapses or clefts between the axon and dendrite. The synapses have chemicals in the axon nerve endings. These chemicals allow communication between the neurons. Hypnosis and biofeedback can disrupt pain signal transmission. Injections can also inhibit transmission of pain signals from the arms or legs to the brain. Chemicals are transferred between nerve synapses which cause transmission of pain signals. Pain signals may be blocked if the chemicals are inhibited from passing from one nerve to another. Pain signals on the way to the brain cross to the opposite side from the location of the injury and therefore, travel to the opposite side of the brain. The pain impulses will then proceed upwards to go to the brain cortex.

It is important to know that pain signals can be dampened by structures and chemicals that exist in the spinal cord. Pain signals enter the spinal cord, then cross to the other side of the spinal cord and proceed upward toward the brain. Pain impulses on the right side go to the left side of the brain. Transduction is a process where electrical signals originate in the nerve endings throughout the body. These impulses are chemically, mechanically and/or thermally mediated and transmitted to the spinal cord where they can be modulated and then sent to the brain. Tissue injury or disease (including arthritis) causes the body to release biochemicals called prostaglandins. Prostaglandins themselves do not cause pain. Prostaglandins do, however, sensitize pain receptors to other chemicals in the body, which facilitate the transmission of pain impulses. Nonsteroidal drugs like ibuprofen decrease the number of prostaglandins produced in the body and may result in a decrease in pain perception. Topical creams such as Ben Gay can decrease the process of transduction at the nerve endings. Transmission is a process where pain signals are transported to the spinal cord. Nerves in body tissues transmit impulses to the spinal cord. Nerve blocks with anesthetics like Novocain can interrupt the transmission of pain impulses to the spinal cord. Once pain impulses reach the spinal cord, they are modulated or changed by other chemicals and nerves that inhibit or lessen the number of pain impulses from going up the spinal cord to the brain. Fibers called internuncial fibers are present within the spinal cord that can decrease pain transmission. The brain can send impulses back to these pain control fibers within the spinal cord to decrease the number of impulses that reach the pain perception center of the brain. This is the basis of hypnosis. Severe pain, however, over-whelms the nerve fibers and hypnosis essentially becomes ineffective. The spinal cord acts like a transformer to intensify or decrease the intensity of pain impulses. Narcotics and anticonvulsants can modulate pain impulses within the spinal cord. In general, the greater the tissue trauma, the more pain transmitting chemicals are produced and the worse the pain.

Chemicals in the central nervous system include bradykinin, substance P, acetylcholine, serotonin and histamine. These chemicals act at the nerve endings and ultimately travel to the spinal cord and brain. GABA (gamma-amino butyric acid) in the spinal cord decreases the number of pain impulses that reach the brain. GABA therefore inhibits pain impulse transmission. Norepinephrine and serotonin are two more chemicals in the spinal cord which attenuate the number of pain impulses, which reach the brain as well. The brain and spinal cord further regulate pain by the production of naturally occurring narcotic-like substances that decrease pain transmission in specific areas of the brain. These narcotic-like drugs are called enkephalins, dynorphins and beta-endorphins. Some of these substances also decrease pain transmission in the spinal cord. Enkephalins inhibit pain at the spinal cord. Enkephalins bind to narcotic receptors. When the analgesic receptors are activated, they inhibit pain signals. Dynorphins exist in both the brain and spinal cord but are more prevalent in the brain. Like enkephalins, these substances bind to narcotic receptors in the brain and spinal cord. The natural beta-endorphins in a body exhibit morphine-like activity. Following injury or stress these endorphins are released into the blood stream. Prostaglandins sensitize pain nerve endings to pain producing tissue chemicals. Antidepressant drugs like Elavil or Prozac decrease pain by increasing norepinephrine and serotonin in the spinal cord. Anti-convulsant drugs like Gabitril (tiagabine) in some instances affect GABA levels in a spinal cord act by enhancing GABA blood levels decreases the number of pain signals in your spinal cord that can go to the brain. Narcotic drugs also decrease pain impulse conduction in both the spinal cord and brain. Injections of local anesthetics with steroids can decrease pain in muscle and nerves in the arms, legs and the trunk of the body.

Nociceptive receptors are free nerve endings and respond to heat mechanical and chemical tissue injury. They have their own activation thresholds. With repeated stimulation they become sensitized. This causes nerve transmission following a low intensity noxious stimulus or even after a non-noxious stimulus. This is the basis of hyperalgesia and allodynia causation. Hyperpathia, hyperalgesia and allodynia are three manifestations of central sensitization, a condition in which a higher than necessary degree of activity is triggered in the central nervous system. Generally, this activity is triggered by nociception, or the nervous system's normal response to painful stimuli. The central nervous system is comprised of the brain and spinal cord, and the function of the central nervous system is to take information in from the outside, for example, hot or cold sensations, or sensations about the position your body is in, process it, and then issue a movement response to it. The word hyperpathia describes an exaggerated reaction to stimuli. In other words, with hyperpathia, your reaction to a stimulus, especially a repeating one, is increased. Such stimuli include touch, vibration, pinpricks, heat, cold, and pressure. A patient's pain threshold is increased, as well.

When a patient has hypopathia, he or she may find that they identify and/or locate the painful stimulus erroneously, or there may be a delay between when he or she comes into contact with the stimulus and when it is experienced. The pain may radiate, and there may be some aftereffects, as well. And it may have an explosive quality to it. Hyperpathia lowers a patient's pain threshold, the sensitivity to things they physically feel. It is similar to hyperalgesia, with the addition that the feeling of pain continues even after the stimulus that causes it has been removed. To understand hyperpathia, begin with hyperalgesia, as this is a predominant type of neuropathic pain, and often accompanied by hyperalgesia. Hyperalgesia is an augmented pain response. In other words, with hyperalgesia, there is increased pain response to a painful stimulus. Your pain threshold may be lowered, as well. Allodynia is central sensitization pain response to stimuli that normally does not provoke pain. For example, for most people, stroking a cat is a pleasurable experience. It is not associated to the feeling of pain. But in cases of allodynia, that same action of petting a dog may cause hand pain.

The three major nociceptors in the body are mechano-receptors which respond to pinch and pan park, silent nociceptors that respond to inflammation, and mechanical heat recent receptors which respond to pressure temperature and neurochemical mediators such as histamine, capsaicin and bradykinin. Polly modo receptors are the most common. Alpha beta afferent nerve fibers transmit non noxious stimulus and Alpha Delta and C fibers transmit painful stimuli.   Nerve conduction velocity is dependent on the diameter and the degree of myelination of the nerve axon. Larger nerves have improved electrical conduction. Visceral nociceptors in the abdomen respond to chemical or mechanical stimuli such as distention, ischemia and inflammation. The C fibers can cross the spinal cord to the opposite dorsal horn. As a result, pain is perceived in the midline and one perceives dull and aching sensations. These fibers travel with sympathetic nerve fibers.

These nociceptors transmit impulses to the spinal cord between T1 and L2. As a result, pain is associated with abnormal sympathetic activities such as nausea vomiting, and he found it kind of makeshift. The celiac plexus is anterior to the vertebral body of L and S one and also carries nociceptive afferent fibers and the sympathetic innervation for the abdominal viscera. The superior hypogastric plexuses are anterior to L5 and carries nociceptive and sympathetic innervation for the large intestine for the pelvic viscera. The ganglionic impar is located on the anterior surface of the coccyx and is the afferent and sympathetic intervention for the pelvic viscera. The stellate ganglia are anterior to C7 and carries afferent and sympathetic innervation to portions of the ipsilateral head neck and arm. The ganglion is anterior to C 7. The transformation of pain starts with activation of the first order neurons that enter the dorsal horn of the spinal cord by way of the dorsal spinal route. A small amount of first order neurons enter the cord from the anterior ventral nerve root. This is the reason why some patients who have rhizotomies for chronic pain continued to feel the pain following the procedure. First order neurons travel up and down several levels in Lissauer's prior to synapsing was second order neurons, then cross and in the spino-thalamic tract and ascend. They cross the midline to the contralateral side.

Second order neurons are nociceptive specific or WDR neurons. Both types receive noxious input from a Delta and c Fibers. Second order neurons synapse with third order neurons in the thalamus and then send impulses through fibers to the internal capsule and to the cerebral cortex. There are both excitatory and inhibitory neurotransmitters. Substance P is an excitatory pain neuropeptide released by first order neurons. Other excitatory transmitters are glutamate, and aspartate which both act on NMDA receptor's and there is CGRP and ATP as well. Both GABA and lysine are important neurotransmitters that are released by inhibitory neurons in the dorsal horn of the spinal cord and they do inhibit pain signals. Glutamate is the main neurotransmitter. GABA b receptor activity plays in important role for analgesia as well. ATP and calcitonin gene peptide are also involved in initiating pain and transmitting pain. Substance P activates NK1 receptors to initiate and transmit pain responses. When Substance P is released blood vessel vasodilation occurs. GABA and glycine are effective in decreasing pain. Injury to the skin can cause two types of hyperalgesia primary and secondary. Primary occurs at the side of injury harm. Secondary hyperalgesia is only triggered by mechanical stimuli while primary is triggered by both mechanical and heat stimuli.

Modern neuroimaging methods (positron emission tomography (PET) and functional MRI (fMRI)) have been used to determine, whether different neuropathic pain symptoms involve similar brain structures. PET studies have suggested that spontaneous neuropathic pain is associated principally with changes in thalamic activity and the medial pain system, which is preferentially involved in the emotional dimension of pain. Fear, suffering and pain are in different areas of the brain, but these areas are connected to each other. These interconnections ultimately can communicate with areas of the brain such as the midbrain that control heart rate and the respiratory rate as well. Aging of the nervous system is characterized by a general loss of neuronal substance. The most obvious sign is a reduced average brain weight in the elderly; brain weight was reported to be 1375 g at age 20 and 1200 g at age 80.

The number of peripheral neurons also decreases, and muscles become innervated by fewer axons, possibly leading to denervation atrophy. A particular neuromuscular junction, however, is not functionally changed with aging. Nerve conduction velocity is slightly affected by aging and tends to become slower in elderly individuals. The overall loss of neuronal substance and decreased synaptic activity may be one explanation for the higher susceptibility of the elderly to drugs that interact with the peripheral or central nervous system. Mental capacity does show a decrease in middle age (45) and a steeper drop after 65, but individual variation is great and appears somewhat dependent on how much mental stimulation one receives. The same principle applies to memory.

Memory loss more often affects short-term memory rather than long-term memory. Usual aging is accompanied by a lower production of neurotransmitters, but only when the drop approaches 50%, will dementia ensue. About 15% of the elderly have severe dementia. If the dementia is the result of acute electrolyte imbalances of sodium or potassium, thyroid dysfunction, drug toxicity or illness, it can be reversed upon treatment of the causal factor. It is extremely difficult to assess pain in patients with dementia. Pain sensation is also decreased in elderly individuals. Several studies have demonstrated that elderly patients have an increased sensitivity to opioid analgesics. It was determined by electroencephalography (EEG) that the most important difference is an increase in the sensitivity in the elderly subject compared to the younger person. In other words, compared to young patients, elderly patients will need lower opioid concentrations for an equal analgesic effect and lower loading doses for equal plasma levels. Elderly individuals will eliminate opioids from their bodies more slowly than young subjects. Pain tolerance is the ability of the individual to handle pain. The pain threshold is the maximum level of pain that a person can tolerate.

The pain threshold in the elderly is higher than in younger patients. This observation may be due to degenerative nerve disease in elderly patients. Elderly women experience more pain than aging men. Pain tolerance may, nevertheless, be decreased in both male and female elderly patients. At high levels of pain intensity, interference decreased with age, although the age by pain intensity interaction effect was small. This evidence converges with aging theories, including socioemotional selectivity theory, which posits that as people age, they become more motivated to maximize positive emotions and minimize negative ones. The results highlight the importance of studying the mechanisms older adults use to successfully cope with pain.

Psychosocial factors associated with shortened telomeres are also common in chronic pain. There is a link between premature cellular aging and chronic pain. Chronic pain is a more serious condition than has typically been recognized in terms of bodily aging. Stressful events in childhood are associated with shorter telomere length in middle-aged men and that part of this relation is explained by depressive mood and low-grade inflammation. Chronic pain conditions are characterized by significant individual variability complicating the identification of pathophysiological markers. Leukocyte telomere length, a measure of cellular aging, is associated with age-related disease onset, psychosocial stress, and health-related functional decline. Psychosocial stress has been associated with the onset of chronic pain and chronic pain is experienced as a physical and psychosocial stressor. Although cognitive ability, walking speed, lung function and grip strength all decline with age, they do so independently of telomere length shortening.

Unfortunately, not unlike ancient times, the diagnosis and

treatment of many chronic painful conditions today remain mostly guesswork in both young and elderly patients. Pain medicine is, for the most part, subjectively based, because pain is a subjective symptom while other medical specialties are based upon objective curative evidence. Pain in general is not bad. Pain is a protective mechanism that warns a patient that the body has something wrong in some location. The International Association for the Study of Pain defines pain as" an unpleasant sensory and emotional experience associated with tissue injury as a result of trauma (e.g. bone fracture) or disease (e.g. cancer, shingles). Pain has psychological effects in some instances especially when pain is severe. Pain may cause anxiety and depression. Acute pain is associated with injury, bone fractures, surgery or sprains and strains. Once these entities have healed sometimes, the pain continues. Arthritis is another example of chronic pain.

Arthritic pain is caused by continuous joint destruction. However, once the pain becomes chronic, it becomes problematic. Not only does pain become a personal problem but pain can become a social problem with creation of family problems, loss of self-esteem and lost wages. Fibromyalgia patients have alterations in CNS anatomy, physiology, and chemistry that potentially contribute to the symptoms experienced by these patients. Studies were previously done that investigated the impact of age and gender on (1) experimental pressure pain detection thresholds and pressure pain tolerance thresholds and (2) participants' self-reports of pain intensity and unpleasantness at supra threshold and subthreshold levels.

The intensity and unpleasantness of the pain stimulus were significantly rated lower in the elderly as compared with the young. No gender differences were observed in the report of intensity and unpleasantness of the stimulations. The elderly appraise pain experiences using different psychological strategies. Pain impulses are, in essence, electrical signals that travel from various areas of the body such as the extremities, heart, appendix, etc. to the spinal cord and eventually reach the brain where the pain signals are processed like data in a computer.   The brain is like a computer hard drive, which stores painful experiences that ultimately result in the suffering associated with chronic pain. Pain is produced by unpleasant stimuli to nerve endings throughout the body which include chemical, extreme heat cold and mechanical injury. These nerve endings are silent until mechanical, heat or cold injures tissue occur. As people age, they become more motivated to maximize positive emotions and minimize negative ones. The results highlight the importance of studying the mechanisms older adults use to successfully cope with pain.

A nerve is composed of neurons. A neuron is an electrically excitable cell in the nervous system that processes and transmits information to the brain and spinal cord. A neuron has one axon that takes nerve signals away from the neuron. The long end of the axon communicates with multiple dendrites. Neurons are the significant core components of the brain and spinal cord as well as peripheral nerves. Neurons are typically composed of a cell body, a dendrite and an axon. Neurons receive input from dendrites and transmit output via the axon. Neurons are the building blocks of nerves. In other words, multitudes of neurons are necessary to form a nerve. Nerves that exist outside of the central nervous system are called a ganglion.

The stellate ganglion in the neck is an example. An injection into this ganglion may relieve pain associated with Reflex Sympathetic Dystrophy (now called Complex Regional Pain Syndrome). Various ganglia may form a plexus. An example of a plexus is your celiac plexus. Sometimes this plexus is blocked with numbing medicine, phenol or alcohol to relieve severe abdominal pain. Action potentials generated by the neuron initiate pain signals. If the skin is pinched a mechanical pain receptor initiates an action potential. An action potential begins after a depolarization such that it could cause a membrane transitory modification, turning prevalently permeable to sodium ions more than to potassium ions. Sodium permeability can cause an action potential. A neuropathy generates a local accumulation of sodium channels, with a consequent increase of density. This model seems to be the basis of neuron hyper excitability. Calcium channels have also an important role in cell function. An intra-cellular calcium increase contributes to depolarization processes, through kinase and determines the phosphorylation of membrane proteins that can make powerful the efficacy of the channels them-selves. Following an acute injury, AMPA receptors are stimulated, which cause sharp pain. Receptors (areas in the body where biochemicals or drugs attach) are present in the spinal cord are called NMDA (N-methyl-D aspartate) receptors and cause chronic pain. When these NMDA receptors are stimulated, pain becomes more severe and this extreme pain is maintained, which implies that the pain does not decrease.

The Rexed laminae represent a system of organizing the neurons of the spinal cord. They are named after Dr. Bror Rexed who was a Swedish neuroscientist. There are ten Rexed laminae and they roughly follow a topographic organization, with the lower numbers (I, II) being towards the posterior spinal cord and the higher numbers (IX, X) being towards the front of the spinal cord. Layer I contain neurons that receive pain and temperature information from the body and limbs via the axons coming from the dorsal root ganglia of the spinal cord. The neurons in layer I then pass this information along to the brain via the spinothalamic tract on the opposite side of the cord. Layer II, which is also known as the substantia gelatinosa, gets information from the spinothalamic tract as well as the dorsal spinal columns. The spinothalamic tract relays information about painful stimuli and the dorsal columns relay information about non-painful stimuli. Therefore, the neurons in layer two receive information about both painful and non-painful stimuli. These neurons then send information to Rexed laminae III and IV. The neurons in these laminae then pass the sensory information to the brain where it is further interpreted.

Interestingly, there are large amounts of opiate responsive neurons in laminae II of the spinal cord. The nucleus proprius, aka, layers III and IV, receives information from the body about touch and proprioception (hence the name "proprius"). It then relays this information to numerous areas in the brainstem, brain, and other Rexed laminae for further processing. Layer V receives information from a wide variety of sources including pain sensation from the bodies' organs, as well as information about movement from the brain (via the corticospinal tracts) and brainstem (via the rubrospinal tracts). The VI layer can be divided into two sections: medial and lateral. The medial layer gets input from muscle spindles. Muscle spindles (by way of type Ia fibers) communicate to the spinal cord concerning how much a given muscle is being stretched. The neurons in the medial layer act as messengers for this information. The lateral layer gets information from the brain and brainstem via multiple descending tracts. The neurons in this layer send information to two places: the cerebellum (via the ventral spinocerebellar tracts) and motor neurons in the anterior horn of the spinal cord.

The cerebellum interprets the information and modulates movement and muscle tone accordingly. The direct communication between the neurons in Rexed laminae VI and the motor neurons in the anterior horns are responsible for spinal reflexes. Layer VII is most prominent between the C8 and L2 vertebral bodies. This prominence is known as the dorsal nucleus of Clarke. The neurons in Clarke's nucleus receive lower extremity position and sensory information and then pass that information to the cerebellum via the dorsal spinocerebellar tract.

Layer VII also receives and sends information from and to the bodies' organs. The sympathetic and parasympathetic autonomic system have their pre-ganglionic neurons in Rexed laminae VII. These neurons are responsible for the fight or flight response (sympathetic) and rest and digest (parasympathetic) functions of the bodies' organs. Neurons in layer VIII obtain information from the reticulospinal and vestibulospinal tracts. The reticulospinal tract is important in maintaining the tone of muscles that flex joints. The vestibulospinal system helps maintain muscles that are important in extending joints. This layer contains the α, β, and γ motor neurons of the cord. Simply stated, these neurons send impulses to muscles leading to movement. The more complex story is that motor neurons in layer IX are influenced by numerous inputs from other Rexed laminae, as well as by descending information coming from the brain. The neurons in layer IX are topographically organized based on what type of muscle (flexor or extender) they control, as well as where in the body that muscle is located (axial or limb).

Neurons that are located towards the center of the cord control axial muscles and those located towards the periphery of the cord control the muscles of the limbs. No one really knows what layer X actually does. In summary, The Rexed laminae are layers of neurons within the spinal cord that perform specific functions. In general, neurons in the laminae towards the back of the cord are predominately involved in interpreting and relaying sensory information from the body to the brain. On the other hand, neurons in the laminae towards the front of the cord are involved primarily in executing movement and controlling the functions of the body's organs.

The brain is responsible for the suffering associated with pain. Pain results in bodily responses, especially with respect to the cardiovascular system (heart rate increases, blood pressure increases, renal arteries constrict, etc.). When pain is severe, the brain can cause the body to increase both the heart rate and blood pressure. Extreme pain can also result in profuse sweating as well as nausea and vomiting. There are different types of nerve endings throughout the body. The pain nerve endings become hyper excitable when stimulated by injury, inflammation or a tumor. Occasionally, the nerve endings remain irritable even after the painful stimulus has been removed.

Pain signals from areas in the body reach the brain by four processes (transduction, transmission, modulation and perception). Axons carry pain fibers away from the neuron and direct them to the dendrites of the next neuron until they terminate in the brain or spinal cord. Remember that the axons and dendrites do not touch. They form synapses or clefts between the axon and dendrite. The synapses have chemicals in the axon nerve endings. These chemicals allow communication between the neurons.

References

1. Calvino, B., Grilo, R.M. (2006) Central pain control. Joint Bone Spine; 73: 1, 10-16.

2. Farquhar-Smith, P. (2007) Anatomy, physiology and pharmacology of pain. Anaesthesia and Intensive Care Medici

8. OPOIDS

An opioid crisis exists in the United States today. An opiate
is a product such as morphine and codeine historically derived
from the juice of Papaver somniferous, the opium poppy. An
opioid, on the other hand, is a compound that possesses
morphinelike characteristics but may not necessarily be derived
from the juice of Papaver somniferum. Codeine itself, has no
intrinsic analgesic effect but requires a metabolic step to occur
(which converts it to morphine) for analgesia to be produced.
In the initial phases of RA, pain results from inflammation, as
evidenced by tenderness and swelling of the joint as well as
laboratory findings (e.g., increased C-reactive protein, anemia,
thrombocytosis). "Opioid" is the term used to refer to a group of
substances that have the analgesic and other properties of
morphine. This includes the naturally occurring opiates,
semisynthetic opiates, and endogenous opioids.

The term "opiate" was initially used to denote any derivative
of the poppy plant. As synthetic and semisynthetic products
became available and endogenous peptides with morphine like
activity were identified, it became clear that the term had to be
modified. It still holds some of its literary significance as any
substance capable of assuaging suffering. Opioids have been the
mainstay of treatment of moderate to severe pain in patients
with cancer and in many acute pain syndromes. Although many
patients with chronic noncancer pain have been successfully

treated with opioids, their role in chronic pain of noncancer origin is still being defined. In the 1960s and 1970s, opioid treatment was considered the antithesis of good treatment for chronic pain of noncancer origin. In the 1980s and 1990s, it gained greater acceptance.

For treatment of both cancer and noncancer chronic pain, there are few true long-term studies to help practitioners fully understand the potential benefits and risks of such therapy. In recent years, guidelines have been established for the safe and efficacious use of opioids in the treatment of many noncancer pain syndromes. The guidelines suggest that opioid therapy for chronic noncancer pain should be considered only after other reasonable attempts at analgesia have failed. A history of substance abuse or severe character pathology should be considered relative contraindications. One practitioner should manage the prescribed opiates, and he or she must be experienced in their use and able to recognize and deal with adverse reactions such as cognitive impairment, constipation, and aberrant use. The potential risks and benefits should be discussed with the patient and clearly documented in the patient file.

"Narcotic" is now a term that has more legal implications than it does pharmacologic ones. It was initially used to denote any drug capable of producing narcosis. It was generally applied to the opiates. However, the term is now used to denote drugs of abuse that are controlled by government agencies. The old name for one of the federal agencies was the Bureau of Narcotics and Dangerous Drugs. Currently, the main regulatory agency on a national level is the Drug Enforcement Agency. The term opioid is now preferred instead of narcotic when describing opioid analgesics. Morphine and codeine are two of the most widely used naturally occurring opioid alkaloids. Morphine is the prototype of the opioid drug. It binds primarily to mu receptors, producing analgesia and respiratory depression. Opioid analgesia is thought to be mediated through a direct interaction with an opioid receptor. Thus far, the opioid receptors responsible for analgesia have been identified in the spinal cord, the brainstem, and the cerebral cortex.

It is less clear at present what analgesic role is played by the opiate receptors that have been identified in the peripheral nervous system. The weak analgesics have a ceiling effect. This implies that there is a dosing level after which side effects accrue more rapidly than analgesic effects. The potent opioids have no such ceiling. As tolerance develops or disease progresses, the doses can be increased. Codeine is one of the most commonly used weak opioids. As doses escalate, nausea and constipation limit efficacy. For example, though 30 mg of codeine provides more analgesia than 15 mg, and 60 mg provides more than 30 mg, etc., higher doses are limited by side effects.

Oxycodone is often listed as a weak opioid. However, this designation is mainly a function of the acetaminophen or aspirin with which it is commonly combined, and in reality, oxycodone by itself is likely more potent than morphine. When used as a single agent and not in combination with another agent, oxycodone can be given in increasing doses, without as clear a ceiling. Morphine is the prototype of the potent group, against which other opioids have been judged despite the fact that other commonly prescribed drugs, including hydrocodone and oxycodone, are more potent than morphine. Morphine is a relatively short serum half-life drug (2 to 3 hours), as is hydromorphone. Methadone, another potent opioid, has a much longer terminal serum half-life, potentially extending to 54 hours; however, its analgesic serum half-life is often much shorter (6 to 8 hours, for example). Prescribing methadone in particular can be very challenging as a result because increasing the dose too quickly can lead to serious and potentially fatal outcomes. The three main opioid subtypes are the mu, kappa, and delta receptors.

From the standpoint of analgesia, the mu receptor seems to be the most important. There may be subtypes of these receptors, with different drugs having different affinities for given receptor subtypes and different patients having different receptor subtypes as well. There also may be analgesic activity at the delta and kappa sites. When a drug combines with a receptor site and produces the action of that receptor, it is considered an agonist. A drug that binds with a receptor and inhibits activity is considered an antagonist. Naloxone is an example of a pure antagonist drug. Semisynthetic and synthetic products have been produced that are both agonist and antagonist at opioid receptors.

The hope in producing these drugs was that they would be agonist for analgesic effects and antagonist for the respiratory depression and sedative effects of the opioids. Examples of mixed agonist-antagonist drugs include pentazocine, butorphanol, and buprenorphine. New preparations of these drugs, specifically buprenorphine, are being or have been developed. The administration of a mixed agonist-antagonist drug to a patient who is physically dependent on an agonist may produce a withdrawal syndrome. The first endogenous opioids to be discovered were the endorphins and enkephalins. These are polypeptides that are synthesized in the brain and spinal cord. They bind with opioid receptors and produce analgesia. Since the discovery of endorphins and enkephalins in the early 1970s, a number of other peptide products have been described. Mixed agonist-antagonist drugs differ from pure agonist analgesics.

Clinically, the most important concept is that these mixed drugs have a ceiling effect. That is, with increasing doses, side effects supervene, and further analgesia cannot be achieved.

When tolerance develops to pure agonist drugs, drug doses can be increased to obtain further analgesia. In patients who are opioid dependent, administration of a mixed agonist-antagonist may precipitate withdrawal. Efficacy refers to the ability of the drug to produce a given response in an appropriate clinical setting. Potency refers either to the number of milligrams required to produce an effect or to the affinity with which a drug binds to a receptor. Thus, a drug may be very potent (able to produce a response at a very low dose) but not have great efficacy (because of intolerable side effects).

Opioids and nonsteroidal anti-inflammatory drugs work at different sites. The opioids combine with the opioid receptor, primarily in the central nervous system. The nonsteroidal anti-inflammatory drugs are cyclooxygenase inhibitors and their primary site of action is in the peripheral nervous system. Most studies done to determine the clinical potency of the opioid analgesics were done against a standard dose of 10 mg of intramuscular morphine. The number of milligrams of a given drug required to produce the same degree of analgesia as 10 mg of morphine is referred to as the "equi analgesic dose." Most opioids are far more potent when given parenterally than orally. To achieve a dose equianalgesic to 10 mg of IM morphine, 20 to 60 mg of hydrocodone would have to be administered orally. This is because of a "first pass" effect in the liver.

Approximately 50% to 80% of an opioid is inactivated by

hepatic metabolism after oral administration. The extent of this first pass effect varies from drug to drug. Hydromorphone, for example, is five times as potent on a milligram basis after IM injection than it is after oral administration. Methadone, on the other hand, has only a 2:1 ratio. The equianalgesic doses of hydromorphone, methadone, Demerol, and levorphanol that would equate with 10 mg of intramuscular morphine would require 1.5 mg of hydromorphone, 10 mg of methadone, and 2 mg of levorphanol. When switching to methadone from another opioid, the calculated dose should be decreased by about 75%. Discrepancies may also exist depending on the direction of the switch (methadone to morphine, or morphine to methadone). The relatively pure opioid agonists include drugs such as morphine, codeine, oxycodone, oxymorphone, levorphanol, fentanyl, and methadone. The mixed agonist-antagonist drugs that are in popular use are pentazocine, butorphanol, and buprenorphine.

Methadone and levorphanol are two of the most commonly used long serum half-life drugs, having a half-life of anywhere from 12 to over 50 hours. With prolonged use, half-life extends markedly. Morphine and hydromorphone are prototypes of the short serum half-life drugs. When used as immediate-release products, morphine and hydromorphone should generally be dosed every 2 to 4 hours. If a sustained-release or controlled-release product is used, morphine can be dosed every 8 to 12 hours. The long serum half-life drugs may have a greater duration of efficacy and can often be dosed every 4 to 6 hours. Despite the long serum half-life, analgesic efficacy does not directly parallel the serum half-life. Patients who are treated with a sustained-release product may have breakthrough pain which is an unexpected increase in pain that was previously well controlled and require intermittent doses of an immediate-release product. It is probably best to use the same medication for the rescue as for the standing dose. It should be offered on an as needed basis every 2 to 3 hours and should be approximately 10% of the total daily dose.

When given by the parenteral route, opioids are anywhere from two to five times as potent on a milligram basis than when given orally. They are also readily absorbed after subcutaneous injection and can be administered intravenously. Rectal and sublingual preparations are also available for some opioids. Fentanyl is available as a transdermal patch. In general, the intramuscular route should be avoided. The injection itself is painful and offers little or no advantage over the subcutaneously or intravenous routes. Fentanyl is a relatively potent opioid analgesic. The application of a transcutaneous patch allows for relatively stable serum levels of fentanyl over 48 to 72 hours. This cuts down the need for repeated dosing and for the pain of parenteral administration. However, after application of the first patch, there is a delay of 12 to 24 hours in achieving adequate analgesia. During this time, rescue doses must be given. Furthermore, if side effects ensue, removal of the patch will not immediately eliminate them because a subcutaneous reservoir of drug has been formed. The dose of drug is directly related to the surface area of the patch. It is available as 12, 25, 50, 75, and 100 micrograms per hour. Direct equianalgesic studies with morphine have not been published, but a 100-micrograms-per-hour patch applied every 72 hours is approximately equianalgesic to 200 mg per day of morphine. The absorption of the fentanyl patch varies with the state of vascular dilatation. Fever or local heat can produce vasodilatation that produces more rapid absorption and systemic distribution of the opioid preparation.

Patients must be cautioned not to apply a heating pad to the area where the patch is applied. Local reactions to the adhesive have also been described. Constipation is the most common and bothersome clinical side effect of the opioids. It is usually defined as a reduction in the frequency of bowel movements to less than one every three days, or difficulty in passing stool. Respiratory depression, tolerance, dependence may also occur. Nausea and vomiting are not uncommon at the start of opioid therapy. However, tolerance usually occurs within days to weeks, and a specific therapy is not usually required. If nausea persists, opioid rotation may be tried, or the route of administration may be changed. There are two circumstances in which respiratory depression may occur unexpectedly. First, when using long serum half-life drugs, remember that five serum half-lives are required to reach steady state. Thus, when using a drug such as methadone or levorphanol, it may require more than a week to achieve steady state.

During this titration period, great care must be taken because serum levels may be escalating despite stable dosing. The second circumstance occurs in patients who undergo a pain-relieving procedure after they have been on large doses of opioids. Patients may tolerate large doses while they are in pain. However, if they undergo radiation therapy, cordotomy, or some other procedure directed at the pain syndrome itself, they may no longer be as tolerant to the opioids. Opioid overdose treatment depends directly on the situation in which the overdose has occurred and the severity of side effects. If there is only somnolence, without respiratory depression, simply cutting back on the dose or holding a few doses is usually enough to reverse the side effects. If there is severe respiratory depression, more urgent measures are required. In these cases, naloxone may be administered intravenously. However, if it is given as a bolus, patients who have been taking opioids chronically may experience withdrawal. Therefore, naloxone should be diluted in 10 ml of saline and administered slowly. Naloxone, however, has a much shorter serum half-life than most opioids. Repeated doses may be required. Tolerance refers to a situation in which decreased effects are noticed despite stable doses of a drug or increasing doses of a drug are required to maintain a given effect. In experimental models, this can develop quite rapidly.

Clinically, however, many patients with stable pain syndromes can be maintained on steady doses of opioids for prolonged periods of time. Physical dependence is a state in which rapid discontinuation of a drug or administration of an antagonist produces an abstinence syndrome. With the opioids, an abstinence syndrome is characterized by abdominal discomfort, borborygmus, goose flesh, nausea, and yawning. In addicted subjects, there is marked drug craving. In nonaddicted subjects, there is simply severe discomfort. Addiction is a biopsychosocial condition in which there is psychological dependence on a drug, preoccupation with securing its supply, use despite harm, use for nonmedical purposes, and a high incidence of recidivism. This is actually quite rare in patients treated appropriately with opioids for pain. Even in patients with pain of nonmalignant origin, opioid addiction is quite uncommon.

Opioid responsiveness is the analgesia that can be achieved from opioids as the dose is titrated to an endpoint defined either by intolerable side effects or the occurrence of acceptable analgesia. By contrast, if side effects impose a limit on dose escalation, the pain is said to be relatively opioid unresponsive. There is always a balance between effects and side effects. A number of factors can influence opioid responsiveness, including the type of pain (neuropathic pain is often relatively unresponsive), the temporal pattern of the pain (incidence of pain may be difficult to control), opioid tolerance or disease progression (may require very high doses), and idiosyncratic patient issues (may limit responsiveness). Strategies to overcome opioid unresponsiveness include more aggressive management of side effects (an attempt to "open the therapeutic window").

If analgesia cannot be obtained with a specific drug, it may make sense to try different opioids. This can be done sequentially, until an appropriate balance is found between analgesia and side effects. As generally used today, patient-controlled analgesia refers to an arrangement whereby patients are able to administer their own drugs on a set basis. Usually this is by the intravenous route. Intravenous access is established, and a system is attached by which the patient may bolus small amounts of opioid every few minutes. A "lockout period" is also established to avoid overdosing. PCA can be done with or without a continuous infusion. This modality is most often used for patients in acute pain settings, such as those experiencing postoperative pain.

References

1. AAPM, APS et al. The use of opioids for the treatment of chronic pain. A consensus statement from the American Academy of Pain Medicine and the American Pain Society. Clinical Journal of Pain. 1997; 13:6–8.

2. Ballantyne JC, Mao J. Opioid therapy for chronic pain. New England Journal of Medicine. 2003; 349:1943–1953.

3. Chou R, Clark E, Helfand M. Comparative efficacy and safety of long-acting oral opioids for chronic non-cancer pain: A systematic review. Journal of Pain and Symptom Management. 2003; 26:1026–1048.

4. Noble M, Tregear SJ, Treadwell JR, Schoelles K. Long-term opioid therapy for chronic noncancer pain: a systematic review and meta-analysis of efficacy and safety. Journal of Pain and Symptom Management. 2008; 35:214–228.

5. Portenoy RK, Foley KM. Chronic use of opioid analgesics in non-malignant pain: Report of 38 cases. Pain. 1986; 25:171–186.

9. NUTRITION IMPROVES ONES SELF BEING

Drugs are chemicals that can interrupt the communication between the neurons. Hypnosis and biofeedback can disrupt pain signal transmission. Injections can also inhibit transmission of pain signals from the arms or legs to the brain. It is important to understand the following processes in order to understand how pain can be treated effectively. Transduction is a process where electrical signals originate in the nerve endings throughout the body. These impulses are chemically, mechanically and/or thermally mediated and transmitted to the spinal cord where they can be modulated and then sent to the brain. Tissue injury or disease (including arthritis) cause the body to release biochemicals called prostaglandins.

Prostaglandins themselves do not cause pain. Prostaglandins do, however, sensitize pain receptors to other chemicals in the body, which facilitate the further transmission of pain impulses. Nonsteroidal drugs like ibuprofen decrease the number of prostaglandins produced in the body and may result in a decrease in pain perception. Topical creams such as Ben Gay can decrease the process of transduction at the nerve endings. Transmission is a process where pain signals are transported to the spinal cord. Nerves in body tissues transmit impulses to the spinal cord. Nerve blocks with anesthetics like Novocain can interrupt the transmission of pain impulses to the spinal cord. Once pain impulses reach the spinal cord, they are modulated or changed by chemicals and nerves that inhibit or lessen the number of pain impulses from going up the spinal cord to your brain. Fibers called internuncial fibers are present within the spinal cord that can decrease pain transmission. The brain can send impulses back to these pain control fibers within the spinal cord to decrease the number of impulses that reach the pain perception center of the brain. This is the basis of hypnosis. Severe pain, however, over-whelms the nerve fibers and hypnosis essentially becomes ineffective. The spinal cord acts like a transformer to intensify or decrease the intensity of pain impulses. Narcotics and anticonvulsants can modulate pain impulses within the spinal cord. Finally, pain impulses reach the brain.

In summary, a stimulus (pin prick) produces a response (pain perception). When a stimulus produces, tissue injury, chemicals are released at the site of nerve injury, which cause pain fibers to become hyperactive. These chemicals include bradykinin, histamine, substance p, acetylcholine, serotonin and histamine. These chemicals further act at the nerve endings and ultimately travel to the spinal cord and brain. GABA (gamma-amino butyric acid) in the spinal cord decreases the number of pain impulses that reach the brain. GABA inhibits pain impulse transmission. Norepinephrine and serotonin are two more chemicals in the spinal cord which attenuate the number of pain impulses, which reach the brain. The brain and spinal cord regulate pain by the production of naturally occurring narcotic-like substances that decrease pain transmission in specific areas of the brain. These narcotic-like drugs are called enkephalins, dynorphins and beta-endorphins. Enkephalins inhibit pain at the spinal cord. Enkephalins bind to narcotic receptors. When the analgesic receptors are activated, they inhibit pain signals.

Dynorphins exist in both the brain and spinal cord but are more prevalent in the brain. Like enkephalins, these substances bind to narcotic receptors in the brain and spinal cord. The natural beta-endorphins in a body exhibit morphine-like activity. Following injury or stress these endorphins are released into the blood stream. Prostaglandins sensitize pain nerve endings to pain producing tissue chemicals. Antidepressant drugs like Elavil or Prozac decrease pain by increasing norepinephrine and serotonin in the spinal cord.

Anti-convulsant drugs like Gabitril (tiagabine) in some instances affect GABA levels in a spinal cord act by enhancing GABA blood levels decreases the number of pain signals in the spinal cord that can go to the brain. Narcotic drugs also decrease pain impulse conduction in both the spinal cord and brain. Injections of local anesthetics with steroids can decrease pain in muscle and nerves in the arms, legs and the trunk of the body. Patients may report combinations of spontaneous pain evoked by stimuli that normally induce no/little sensation of pain. Modern neuroimaging methods (positron emission tomography (PET) and functional MRI (fMRI)) have been used to determine, whether different neuropathic pain symptoms involve similar brain structures. PET studies have suggested that spontaneous neuropathic pain is associated principally with changes in thalamic activity and the medial pain system, which is preferentially involved in the emotional dimension of pain. Fear, suffering and pain are in different areas of the brain, but these areas are connected to each other. These interconnections ultimately can communicate with areas of the brain such as the midbrain that control heart rate and the respiratory rate as well.

Aging of the nervous system is characterized by a general loss of neuronal substance. The most obvious sign is a reduced average brain weight in the elderly; brain weight was reported to be 1375 g at age 20 and 1200 g at age 80. The number of peripheral neurons also decreases, and muscles become innervated, overall, by fewer axons, possibly leading to denervation atrophy. A particular neuromuscular junction is not functionally changed with aging. Nerve conduction velocity is slightly affected by aging and tends to become slower in elderly individuals. The overall loss of neuronal substance and decreased synaptic activity may be one explanation for the higher susceptibility of the elderly to drugs that interact with the peripheral or central nervous system. Several studies have demonstrated that elderly patients have an increased sensitivity to opioid analgesics. It was determined by electroencephalography (EEG) that the most important difference is an increase in the sensitivity in the elderly subject compared to the younger person. In other words, compared to young patients, elderly patients will need lower opioid concentrations for an equal analgesic effect and lower loading doses for equal plasma levels. Elderly individuals will eliminate opioids from their bodies more slowly than young subjects. Pain tolerance is the ability of the individual to handle pain. Pain threshold is the maximum level of pain that a person can tolerate. The pain threshold in the elderly is higher than in younger patients. This observation may be due to degenerative nerve disease in elderly patients. Elderly women experience more pain than aging men. Pain tolerance may, nevertheless, be decreased in both male and female elderly patients.

It is important that elderly patients realize the adverse effects of numerous environmental factors, including improperly balanced diets which may accelerate the onset of ailments related to the climacteric period. A study was done to examine the relationships between diets and the quality of life of working women aged 50-64 years. Analysis of the effect of a healthy diet on the quality of life showed that statistically significant correlations were observed in the case of mental health, functioning in society, emotionality, vitality, and well-being.

Reference

1. Rocz Panstw Zakl Hig.

    ftp://wydawnictwa.pzh.gov.pl/roczniki_pzh/(2):169-175.

    Relationships between diets and the quality of life to

    women aged 50 to 64, Stępień E1, Baj-Korpak J1,

    Gawlik K1, Bergier B1, Pocztarska A1, Sidor M1,

    Szepeluk A1.

10. PLASTICITY

Pain can result from nerve damage to either the peripheral or the central nervous system. Traditionally, abnormal pain from peripheral nerves has been termed 'neuropathic' and pain from damage to central nerves in the brain and spinal cord has been called 'central pain'. However, in clinical practice, the symptoms and signs can be the same for both conditions and it is not always easy to tell where the injury is occurring. The nervous system has the ability to adapt to injury and can change its response to stimulation. The pathways described above are not hard-wired, but instead display the phenomenon of plasticity. Several mechanisms to explain how these changes take place have been proposed and some are summarized below. When an A delta or C fiber is cut or partially damaged (e.g. in post- herpetic neuralgia), it tries to repair itself. In doing so it does not heal in its original form but instead a neuroma, or swelling, develops around the joined axon. Spontaneous electrical activity can be seen around neuromata, thought to be due to altered distribution, expression and gating properties of sodium channels. Ectopic impulse generation can also be seen at the spinal cord level in dorsal root ganglia. In addition, peripheral nociceptors become sensitized by injury so that they: have a lower threshold for firing and can increase their response to noxious stimuli can fire in response to non-noxious stimuli.

Damaged nerves become the foci of hyper-excitability and

ectopic discharge. Ectopic firing is influenced by physical stimuli (e.g. heat or cold) and the metabolic and chemical environment of the nerve. Injury also causes changes in the Schwann cells and glia that surround axons. These are non-neuronal cells that provide support and nutrition to nerves. Injury causes phenotypic shifts leading to changes in growth factor, breakdown of the myelin sheaths surrounding nerves and a resultant change in axonal function. Furthermore, uninjured axons can spread into areas of injury and, particularly if this involves central neurons, the result is the spread of pain to uninjured areas and development of 'mirror' pain.

The sympathetic nervous system can play a role in some painful conditions, such as complex regional pain syndrome. It is responsible for both causing and maintaining the pain. Injury to a limb can cause abnormal processing of information in the spinal cord, which in turn leads to abnormal sympathetic outflow to the injured extremity. The result is neuropathic pain, which is often resistant to treatment and the following changes in the limb: abnormal regulation of vasculature, edema, discoloration, changes in sweating, temperature changes, trophic changes in skin, reduced motor activity in the affected part. Primary afferents from nociceptors can be influenced by sympathetic neurons. The sympathetic postganglionic neuro- transmitter, noradrenaline can exert its effect anywhere along the pathway from the free nerve endings to the dorsal root ganglion. In response to injury, nociceptor neurons can show increased expression of a-adrenoceptors, making them more responsive to the chemical influence of noradrenaline. In addition, sympathetic terminals sprout into the dorsal root ganglia (DRG) after nerve injury and may come into contact with sensory neurons here. Alteration of the blood supply to afferent nerve terminals may also contribute to their sensitivity to the effects of sympathetic stimulation. Central sensitization happens when changes occur in the dorsal horn of the spinal cord after nerve injury. Repetitive C fiber activation by noxious stimuli leads to a prolonged dorsal horn response. This phenomenon has been termed 'wind-up'.

Within the dorsal horn there is a reduction in local inhibition by the neurotransmitter's GABA and glycine and evidence of excitotoxic death of inhibitory interneurons. At the same time there is a strengthening of excitatory synaptic connections. Incoming axons develop ectopic activity and output to the spinothalamic tract neurons is increased. This process involves neurochemical changes mediated via N-methyl-D-aspartate (NMDA), neurokinins, and nitric oxide. The result of all of these changes is that the sensory threshold for pain signaling is lowered and there is spread of the receptive field. In addition, it has been shown that structural neural rewiring occurs in the dorsal horn of the spinal cord in response to injury. C fiber terminations in the substantia gelatinosa (lamina II) degenerate and Ab (fine touch) fibers, which are usually located in laminae III and IV, sprout into lamina II. This may explain allodynia, where light touch is perceived as painful. These changes seem to be triggered by loss of nerve growth factor. Finally, there are changes at a supraspinal level. Following injury there is evidence of cortical remapping and reorganization in both the primary somatosensory and motor cortices and in the subcortical areas. This is well recognized following limb amputation where lack of afferent input from the amputated limb leads to less occupation of the corresponding area of the somatosensory cortex. As a result, the neighboring cortical area (representing a different anatomical site) expands. The clinical manifestation of these changes is that the patient not only develops phantom limb pain very soon after amputation, but also that the phantom limb can sometimes be mapped out by touching a very different site of their body (e.g. pain in phantom hand felt by touching side of face).

A reduction in the intensity of the phantom limb pain by effective treatment can be shown to reverse the cortical changes. Pain usually occurs when the nerves relay a pain signal following an injury or damage somewhere in the body. Neuropathic pain results from damage to the nerves themselves. Uncovering the cause of nerve damage is the first step in treating neuropathic pain. Factors that often cause or contribute to neuropathic pain include cancer, compression of a nerve or nerves, diabetes, excessive alcohol use, hormonal disorders, immune system disorders, Infections, vitamin deficiencies. Unfortunately, the cause of neuropathic pain cannot always be determined or reversed. Receiving care as soon as possible may help prevent or lessen problems that often accompany neuropathy, such as depression, sleeplessness, and diminished functioning. Neuropathy takes many forms, and the treatments for neuropathic pain are varied as well. Diabetes is the most common etiology of polyneuropathy. Treating the underlying issue may stabilize the condition, reducing symptoms. This could involve better blood sugar control in people with diabetic neuropathy to reduce symptoms and prevent additional damage to the nerves. If a vitamin deficiency is causing the pain, changes in diet or supplementation will typically be recommended. Nerves can be compressed at any point, leading to pain. The pressure could be from a herniated disc, a trapped median nerve in a carpal tunnel syndrome, or other causes.

Decompression surgery releases the pressure on the nerve, relieving the pain. This treatment is typically effective when a small number of nerves are affected, but not when nerves over a wide area are compressed. The immediate area of injury as well as nearby areas can be affected when a nerve is injured due to a sudden impact. Neuropathic pain caused by an injury to a nerve may improve with time. Exercises to maintain and improve strength and range of motion. People will generally work with increasing levels of resistance and perform stretches to enhance flexibility. Exercise boosts blood circulation, which in turn increases the flow of oxygen. Exercising can also improve mental outlook and help control blood glucose in people with diabetes.

Mobility issues are common with neuropathy, and lack of exercise can lead to weight gain and other problems that make the condition more difficult. Exercise can improve blood circulation, which strengthens nerve tissues by increasing the flow of oxygen. Pain messages travel along the peripheral nervous system until they reach the spinal cord. The gate control theory proposes that there are "gates" on the bundle of nerve fibers in the spinal cord between the peripheral nerves and the brain. These spinal nerve gates control the flow of pain messages from the peripheral nerves to the brain. Many factors determine how the spinal nerve gates will manage the pain signal. These factors include the intensity of the pain message, competition from other incoming nerve messages (such as touch, vibration, heat, etc.), and signals from the brain telling the spinal cord to increase or decrease the priority of the pain signal.

Depending on how the gate processes the signal, the message can be handled in any of the following ways: allowed to pass directly to the brain, altered prior to being forwarded to the brain or prevented from reaching the brain (by nerve blocks. Pain signals causing phantom pain can arise from amputated limbs. The gate control theory provides a framework to explain this by the complex interaction of the structures of the nervous system and the role of the most complex structure known. Strategies discussed with physical and occupational therapists can be applied to everyday life to make neuropathy pain more manageable. An untreated injury can cause permanent damage.

Folic acid deficiencies can cause neuropathic pain. Folic acid may be of benefit in patients with folic acid deficiencies. At 16 weeks, in a supplemented folic acid group, serum levels of folic acid ($p < 0.001$) increased, homocysteine concentrations decreased ($p < 0.001$), with no change in serum vitamin B12 levels. There was a significant increase in sensory sural amplitude ($p < 0.001$), and components of motor nerves, including amplitude ($p = 0.001$) and velocity ($p < 0.001$), but decreased onset latency of peroneal ($p = 0.019$) and tibial ($p = 0.011$) motor nerves.

Reference

1. Neurol Res. 2019 Apr;41(4):364-368. doi: 10.1080/01616412.2019.1565180. Epub 2019 Feb 7. Effect of folic acid supplementation on nerve conduction velocity in diabetic polyneuropathy patients. Mottaghi T1,2, Khorvash F3, Maracy M4, Bellissimo N5, Askari G.

11. SUGAR ADDICTION

The link between sugar and addictive behavior is tied to the fact that, when a person eats sugar, opioids and dopamine are released from the brain. When a certain behavior causes an excess release of dopamine, one feels a pleasurable "high" that people are inclined to re-experience, and so repeat the behavior. In medicine physicians use 'addiction' to describe a tragic situation where someone's brain chemistry has been altered to compel them to repeat a substance or activity despite harmful consequences. Evidence is mounting that too much added sugar could lead to true addiction as well. The link between sugar and addictive behavior is tied to the fact that, when a person eats sugar, opioids and dopamine are released. Dopamine is a neurotransmitter that is a key part of the "reward circuit" associated with addictive behavior. When a certain behavior causes an excess release of dopamine, you feel a pleasurable "high" that you are inclined to re-experience, and so repeat the behavior. As you repeat that behavior more and more, your brain adjusts to release less dopamine. The only way to feel the same "high" as before is to repeat the behavior in increasing amounts and frequency. This is known as substance abuse. "Research shows that sugar can be even more addicting than cocaine," says Cassie Bjork, R.D., L.D., founder of Healthy Simple Life. "Sugar activates the opiate receptors in our brain and affects the reward center, which leads to compulsive behavior, despite the negative consequences like weight gain, headaches, hormone imbalances, and more." "Studies suggest that every time a person eats sweets that individual is reinforcing those neuropathways, causing the brain to become increasingly hardwired to crave sugar, building up a tolerance like any other drug," she adds.

Research on rats from Connecticut College has shown that Oreo cookies activate more neurons in the brain's pleasure center than cocaine does (and just like humans, the rats would eat the filling first). And a 2008 Princeton study found that, under certain circumstances, not only could rats become dependent on sugar, but this dependency correlated with several aspects of addiction, including craving, binging, and withdrawal. Researchers believe that the casual link between sugar and illegal drugs doesn't just make for dramatic headlines. Not only is there truth to it, but they determined the rewards experienced by the brain after consuming sugar are even "more rewarding and attractive" than the effects of cocaine.

Medical addiction changes brain chemistry to cause binging, craving, withdrawal symptoms, and sensitization." "Excess added sugar can do this too, through changes in the same pathways as addiction to amphetamines or alcohol. Sugar addiction could be an even harder habit to break, according to recent evidence about how added sugar affects our stress hormones." Sugar is also much more prevalent, available, and socially acceptable than amphetamines or alcohol, and so harder to avoid. But whether or not sugar is more addictive than cocaine, researchers and nutritionists are in agreement that yes, sugar has addictive properties, and we need to be getting less of it. There is an increasing body of research demonstrating that sugar can stimulate the brain's reward processing center in a manner that mimics what we see with some recreational drugs. In certain individuals with certain predispositions, this could manifest as an addiction to sugary foods."

The World Health Organization (WHO) cautions people to reduce their intake of "free sugars" to less than 10 percent of daily calories since 1989, saying that doing so can lower your risk for being obese, overweight, or experiencing tooth decay. "Free sugars" include both the sugars naturally found in honey and fruit juice, and sugar added to food and drinks. On food labels, added sugars include words such as glucose, corn syrup, brown sugar, dextrose, maltose, and sucrose, as well as many others. on In 2015, they further suggested reducing free sugar intake to less than 5 percent of calories, about 6 teaspoons. In the United States, sugars account for 14 percent of the average person's calorie intake. Most of this comes from beverages, including energy drinks, alcoholic drinks, soda, fruit drinks, and sweetened coffee and teas. Other common sources are snacks. These don't just include obvious perpetrators, like brownies, cookies, doughnuts, and ice cream. You can also find large quantities of added sugar in bread, salad dressing, granola bars, and even fat-free yogurt. High-calorie sweeteners are in over 95 percent of granola bars, cereals, and sugar-sweetened beverages, most often in the form of corn syrup, sorghum, and cane sugar.

The ODPHP 2015-2020 Dietary Guidelines suggest cutting consumption of added sugars to less than 10 percent of calories per day. To help consumers, the Food and Drug Administration has developed a new food label source that lists added sugars separately, which manufacturers were required to use beginning in 2018. Reducing sugar, especially concentrated sugars, not only limits the amount of sugars ingested but also makes less sweet foods seem sweeter. Dopamine is a neurotransmitter that is a key part of the "reward circuit" associated with addictive behavior. When a certain behavior causes an excess release of dopamine, you feel a pleasurable "high" that you are inclined to re-experience, and so repeat the behavior. As you repeat that behavior more and more, your brain adjusts to release less dopamine. The only way to feel the same "high" as before is to repeat the behavior in increasing amounts and frequency. This is known as substance abuse.

"Research shows that sugar can be even more addicting than cocaine," says Cassie Bjork, R.D., L.D., founder of Healthy

Simple Life. "Sugar activates the opiate receptors in our brain and affects the reward center, which leads to compulsive behavior, despite the negative consequences like weight gain, headaches, hormone imbalances, and more." "Studies suggest that every time we eat sweets, we are reinforcing those neuropathways, causing the brain to become increasingly hardwired to crave sugar, building up a tolerance like any other drug," she adds.   Research on rats from Connecticut College has shown that Oreo cookies activate more neurons in the brain's pleasure center than cocaine does (and just like humans, the rats would eat the filling first). A Princeton study found that, under certain circumstances, not only could rats become dependent on sugar, but this dependency correlated with several aspects of addiction, including craving, binging, and withdrawal. re Medical addiction changes brain chemistry to cause binging, craving, withdrawal symptoms, and sensitization. Excess added sugar can do this too, through changes in the same pathways as addiction to amphetamines or alcohol. Sugar addiction could be an even harder habit to break, according to recent evidence about how added sugar affects our stress hormones. Sugar is also much more prevalent, available, and socially acceptable than amphetamines or alcohol, and so harder to avoid.

There is an increasing body of research demonstrating that sugar can stimulate the brain's reward processing center in a manner that mimics what is seen with some recreational drugs. In certain individuals with certain predispositions, this could manifest as an addiction to sugary foods."   The World Health Organization (WHO) has been warning people to reduce their intake of "free sugars" to less than 10 percent of daily calories since 1989, saying that doing so can lower one's risk for being obese, overweight, or experiencing tooth decay. "Free sugars" include both the sugars naturally found in honey and fruit juice, and sugar added to food and drinks. On food labels, added sugars include words such as glucose, corn syrup, brown sugar, dextrose, maltose, and sucrose, as well as many others. are Most of this comes from beverages, including energy drinks, alcoholic drinks, soda, fruit drinks, and sweetened coffee and teas.   Other common sources are snacks. These don't just include obvious perpetrators, like brownies, cookies, doughnuts, and ice cream. A person can also find large quantities of added sugar in bread, salad dressing, granola bars, and even fat-free yogurt. High-calorie sweeteners are in over 95 percent of granola bars, cereals, and sugar-sweetened beverages, most often in the form of corn syrup, sorghum, and cane sugar. Reducing sugar, especially concentrated sugars, not only limits the amount of sugars ingested but also makes fewer sweet foods seem sweeter.

References

1. Gearhardt AN, Brownell KD. Can food and addiction
    change the game? Biol Psychiatry (2013) 73:802–3.
    10.1016/j.biopsych.2012.07.024

2. Lee PC, Dixon JB. Food for thought: reward
    mechanisms and hedonic overeating in obesity. Curr
    Obes Rep. (2017) 6:353–61. 10.1007/s13679-017-0280-
    9

3. Pretlow RA, Corbee RJ. Similarities between obesity in
    pets and children: the addiction model. Br J Nutr.
    (2016) 116:944–9. 10.1017/S0007114516002774

12. NEUROPATHIC PAIN

Nerve damage results from physical trauma or from a wide variety of illnesses, diseases and medical conditions. Common causes of nerve damage, also referred to as neuropathy, include alcoholism, metabolic disorders such as diabetes or celiac disease, autoimmune disorders such as arthritis, cancer treatments, carpal tunnel syndrome, chronic kidney failure, vitamin deficiencies, toxins and infectious diseases. Physical trauma to nerves from injury, herniated disks, prolonged nerve compression and surgery, as well as certain medications and infections that block oxygen to cells can also cause neuropathy. Symptoms include chronic or recurrent numbness, tingling, sensitivity to touch, weakness, pricking sensations, burning pain or sharp pain. Foods can play an integral role in the comprehensive treatment of neuropathic pain.

Nerve damage occurs when the myelin sheath that covers and protects nerves—much like the rubber encasing surrounding electrical wires—deteriorates. The nerves misfire, triggering other nerve cells, which in turn contribute to further excessive nerve cell activity. Vitamin B12 foods can help heal damaged nerves. Foods with vitamin B12 contribute to the repair and maintenance of nerve cells, and particularly the myelin sheath. Foods that contain high levels of vitamin B12 include calf's liver, sardines, snapper, venison, Chinook salmon, lean beef tenderloin, lamb loin, scallops, shrimp and halibut.

Nerve damage occurs when atoms, often called free radicals, interact with cell tissues and cause deterioration of the cells. Free radicals that are synthesized from oxygen are especially egregious. They not only interact with cells tissues, but also create more radicals. Antioxidants are compounds that neutralize free radicals. Various "superfoods" contain high levels of antioxidants. These foods not only heal damaged nerves, but also may help reduce the risk of cancer and immune diseases and slow the effects of aging. Foods that contain high levels of antioxidants include blueberries, raspberries, blackberries, tomatoes, broccoli, red grapes, garlic, spinach, carrots, pomegranates, dark chocolate and green tea, according to Clemson University Cooperative Extension, located in Clemson, South Carolina.

Inflammation results when the body's immune system attempts to protect itself against invading foreign organisms such as bacteria and viruses. White blood cells and other chemicals attack the invaders and destroy them. Sometimes, however, the body's immune response is misguided, and the immune system attacks and destroys its own tissues. Inflammation causes damage to nerves which causes pain in patients. Certain foods reduce inflammation. Foods high in omega-3 fatty acids have anti-inflammatory properties. High omega-3 foods include flaxseeds, walnuts, soybeans, shrimp and tofu as well as cold water fish such as snapper, sardines, salmon, trout, halibut, tuna and cod.

Nerve pain (called neuropathic pain), is one of the more difficult and uncomfortable types of pain. Whether the pain comes from diabetes, shingles, fibromyalgia, chemotherapy, or a host of other causes, this searing, burning, electric shock kind of pain can leave you miserable. Unfortunately, most physicians are still not trained in treating nerve pain and give anti-inflammatory medications like Motrin (which are not effective and kill over 16,500 Americans unnecessarily each year) or narcotics, which are modestly effective.

Many studies have shown that using nutritional support with lipoic acid 300 mg 2x day, Acetyl-L-Carnitine 2,000 mg a day, Inositol (500-1,000 mg a day), and vitamins B6 (50-100 mg a day) and B12 can actually help heal the nerves and decrease or eliminate the pain. Nerves take time to heal, so natural remedies need to be taken for 3-12 months. In the interim, holistic pharmacies can make powerful creams combining multiple medications effective against nerve pain. These creams are rubbed over the painful areas and can be very effective after 1-2 weeks of use. Being rubbed on the skin though, the total dose to the rest of your body is very low, making it largely side effect free! Other medications can also be very effective.

The term "neuropathic pain," or nerve pain, refers to a wide range of problems that cause diseases of, or injury to, the nervous system. It is a category of pain syndromes and not a single problem. Neuropathic pain can come from malfunction of nerves or the brain associated with illness (e.g., diabetes, low thyroid, etc.), infections (e.g., shingles), pinched nerves, nutritional deficiencies (e.g., vitamin B6 and B12), injury (e.g., stroke, tumors, spinal cord injury, and multiple sclerosis), and medication/treatment side effects (e.g., radiation and chemotherapy, AIDS drugs, Flagyl). It is estimated that 50-80% of diabetics will develop some nerve injury with 30-40% of these having painful diabetic neuropathy unless preventive measures are taken such as nutritional support. Neuropathic pain affects approximately 0.6-1.5% of the U.S. population and 25-40% of cancer patients. This represents over two million Americans.

Neuropathies are characterized by pain that is burning, shooting (often to distant areas), or stabbing. It also has an "electric" quality about it. Tingling or numbness (paresthesias) and increased sensitivity with normal touch being painful (allodynia) are also commonly seen. Ongoing pain is often continually present regardless of what the patient does or does not do. In some cases, pain comes in sudden attacks without any apparent trigger. The diagnosis is made predominantly by history and physical examination, as testing often offers little benefit clinically unless the testing is looking for a treatable cause.

In the presence of nerve pain, it is especially important to look for treatable causes. Laboratory testing should include: a blood count (CBC) and an inflammation/sedimentation rate (ESR), thyroid testing with a Free T4 and TSH, Vitamin B12 level, screening for diabetes with a morning fasting blood sugar and a glycosylated hemoglobin (HgBA1C). The medical history should be assessed for excess alcohol use, vitamin deficiencies, hereditary factors, or treatment with medications that can cause nerve injury. A neurological examination may also give an indication of the cause.

Nerve pain is often associated with a process called "pain central sensitization." The nerves and brain are like wires that carry information. When they become over-stimulated with chronic pain, it may make the whole system over-excitable. In these situations, normal touch and other usually comfortable contact can be painful. This is called allodynia. Medications that stimulate the "calming (GABA) receptors" in the brain, such as a number of anti-seizure medications (see below), can help settle the system and further decreases pain.

Postherpetic Neuralgia follows a rash called herpes zoster. Often called shingles, it is caused by the same virus that causes chickenpox. The first time you get chickenpox, the virus remains in your nerve endings even after the chickenpox is gone. This usually causes no problems. If the virus re-activates in one of the nerve endings, however, it causes a rash all along the distribution of the nerve. The rash of herpes zoster is characterized by being painful and being in a line totally on one side of the body. If the pain persists after the rash is gone, continuing for weeks to years (over one year in half of elderly patients), it is called "Postherpetic Neuralgia (PHN)." The pain tends to be burning, electric, or deep and aching.

PHN affects between 500,000 and 1 million Americans, most of whom are elderly. It can severely disrupt one's life, but fortunately can now be effectively treated in most cases. Painful diabetic neuropathy (PDN) is the most common cause of neuropathy. Alterations in sensation are common, and the feet, which are most often affected, may feel both numb and painful at the same time. There are many factors contributing to nerve injury in diabetes, including decreased circulation, accumulation of toxic byproducts, damage from elevated sugars, and nutritional deficiencies. There are also changes in NMDA and opiate receptors.

Research has shown that many people who are labeled as having diabetic neuropathy actually experience neuropathic pain caused by vitamin B6 or B12 deficiency. In addition, the nutrients inositol has been shown to improve nerve function. The nutrients lipoic acid and Acetyl-L-Carnitine have also been shown to be very helpful for diabetic and other nerve pains, but it can take 3-12 months to begin nerve healing.

Neuropathic pain can also be caused by deficiencies of vitamins B12, B1, B6, D, E and zinc. A number of studies have shown that different types of nerve pain can improve by supplementation with high dose B vitamins. Excess vitamin B6 (over 500 mg a day for years), however, can also cause neuropathy. Vitamin D 2,000 units a day was also shown to decrease diabetic neuropathy pain by 47% after 3 months. Hormonal deficiencies, especially an under-active thyroid, can also cause neuropathic as well as muscular pain. A therapeutic trial of thyroid hormone is reasonable for anybody who has the symptoms of low thyroid including fatigue, cold intolerance, achiness, having low body temperatures, or unexplained inappropriate weight gain.

A pinched nerve can cause nerve pain in many places in the body. Two of the more common ones are low back pain from sciatica and pains in the hand and sometimes wrist from carpal tunnel syndrome. Sciatica usually goes away without surgery by using intravenous colchicine (see chapter 14 of Pain Free 1-2-3), and carpal tunnel syndrome usually resolves after 6 to 12 weeks with vitamin B6 (250 mg a day), thyroid hormone, and wrist splints. Reflex Sympathetic Dystrophy (CRPS) usually manifests as horribly severe pain in one hand or foot but can certainly spread elsewhere.

Neuropathic pain occurs biochemically, making it a very fluid system that can often be quickly modified, resulting in pain relief. Many different chemicals (neurotransmitters) in the body may be involved in pain causation, and therefore it is worth trying different types of medications to determine see which one is effective. The antioxidant lipoic acid (300 m2 times a day) has been shown to be helpful in diabetic neuropathy and should be tried in other neuropathies as well.

Reference

1. Costigan M, Scholz J, Woolf CJ. Neuropathic pain: a maladaptive response of the nervous system to damage. Annu Rev Neurosci. 2009;32:1–32

13. DIETARY DEFICIENCIES

Dietary habits are fundamental issues to assess when modulating health and well-being. Many substances, known to be active antioxidants and anti-inflammatory compounds, should serve this fundamental task. Antinociceptive and analgesic natural compounds include flavonoids, terumbone from ginger root, curcuminoids, 3 polyunsaturated fatty acids, and taurine. Furthermore, correct intake of trace elements and minerals is strategic to reduce inflammation-related pain. Osteoarthritis (OA) patients who are overweight or obese report higher levels of pain compared with their normal-weight OA counterparts. Evidence suggests that overweight or obese OA patients also experience pain relief from eating foods high in calories, fat or sugar. Eating to alleviate pain may be problematic because it can lead to additional weight gain, which may contribute to heightened pain.

Recently, attention to the lifestyle of patients has been rapidly increasing in the field of pain therapy, particularly with regard to the role of nutrition in pain development and its management. the role of nutrition and nutraceuticals, microbiome, obesity, soy, omega-3 fatty acids, and curcumin supplementation as key elements in modulating the efficacy of analgesic treatments, including opioids. It is now recognized that patients with chronic pain should undergo nutritional assessment and counseling, which should be initiated at the onset of pain treatment. Some foods and supplements used in personalized treatment will likely improve clinical outcomes of analgesic therapy and result in considerable improvement of patient compliance and quality of life.

A high-protein diet combined with restriction of carbohydrate and salt is furthermore recommended for patients with chronic pain.

Protein contains the amino acids that are critical for many pain control functions, including formation of many neurotransmitters, hormones, muscle, and cartilage. Other components of a chronic pain diet ideally should contain select dietary supplements that help reduce inflammation, control weight, prevent osteopenia and osteoporosis, and regenerate nerve cells. Practitioners are urged to take a dietary history because the majority of chronic pain patients are woefully deficient in protein intake. Clearly, dietary counseling must be a component of chronic pain care. Plant-food supplements have anti-inflammatory effects. Fruits that are high in anthocyanins have shown to be anti- inflammatory. Carotenoids, found in red, yellow, and orange vegetables work via reducing pro-inflammatory pathways and causing a reduction in pain. Other vegetables, including broccoli, cauliflower, cabbage, and bok choy have various amount of a component that also reduces inflammatory pathways and reduce pain. Studies done on green tea extract show that a component in it has strong anti-inflammatory properties. Soy causes suppression of pro-inflammatory cytokines also. Both ginger and turmeric also work through multiple anti-inflammatory pathways and decrease pain.

Opioid treatment also has a profound effect on the endocrine–nutrition system, compounding the necessity of a pain diet. Patients on opioids commonly gain weight and prefer sweet foods. Weight gain may be profound, with some patients doubling their weight within a few years. Opioid use may cause blood sugar levels to be very unstable and may cause hypoglycemia. Opioids also cause a "sugar desire effect" on opioid receptors. Consequently, the combination of severe chronic pain and opioid treatment can cause deranged glucose metabolism in patients and a potent desire to ingest primarily sugars and starches, with little protein or fat intake. Some patients with pain give a history that about 2 hours after eating a carbohydrate load, such as a doughnut, bagel, or glass of fruit juice, their pain will flare. Obesity has been shown to have increased proinflammatory cytokine levels. C-reactive protein specifically is directly related to amount of adipose tissue, which releases leptin to cause activation of the immune system and pro-inflammatory cytokines. A Western diet is one consisting of high intake of red meat, refined sugars, processed food, and saturated fats.

Vitamin D is known to decrease levels of inflammation. The chronic pain population, including those with fibromyalgia, is generally deficient in vitamin D. Pain patients without adequate vitamin D levels tend to stay on opioids twice as long and take twice as much of the drug as patients with appropriate vitamin D levels. According to the Stanford University Medical School, the role of nutrition and its effect on pain is still in the early stages of research. There are several studies however that show certain substances in foods may help with reducing inflammation, improving mood and reducing the sensation of pain. Examples include: Omega-3 fatty acids – This is found in foods such as flaxseed, walnuts, halibut, shrimp and winter squash. Studies suggest that foods high in Omega-3 may reduce migraine headaches, inflammatory pain and pain associated with multiple sclerosis and arthritis. Tryptophan is present in dairy foods such as milk, yogurt, cottage and parmesan cheese, as well as other foods such as sesame, sunflower and pumpkin seeds. Chocolate, oats, bananas, poultry and turkey also have high levels of tryptophan. Tryptophan may be helpful in reducing neuropathic pain and improving sleep. Furthermore, foods high in fiber are effective in preventing constipation which is known to aggravate back pain. Soy-enriched diets may have positive effects in reducing neuropathic pain. Green tea and cherries may also have pain-relieving properties as well.

The evidence for dietary modification to improve chronic pain is immense. Diet and nutritional supplements are important factors in inflammation and pain, and modification of diet in patients with chronic pain should be a part of a comprehensive treatment plan. Obesity is a risk factor for chronic pain, and obese patients have a higher prevalence of chronic pain.

Obesity, deficient nutrient intake, and poor eating behavior are highly prevalent in patients with chronic pain on long-term opioid therapy.

Reference

J Pain Res. 2016; 9: 1179–1189. Published online 2016 Dec 8. doi: 10.2147/JPR.S115068 Combining pain therapy with lifestyle: the role of personalized nutrition and nutritional supplements according to the SIMPAR Feed Your Destiny approach. Manuela De Gregori,

14. GENDER EFFECT

Sex differences in clinical pain are well documented, with women at an increased risk for many chronic pain conditions compared to men. Sex differences in responses to opioids have also been reported, such that women appear to show more significant analgesia in response to morphine and mixed action opioids, but women report greater side effects as well. Various biopsychosocial mechanisms contribute to sex differences in pain and analgesia. Sex differences (i.e., quantitative differences) in which the endpoint exists on a continuum and males and females, on average, differ in their responses. Several prospective studies have indicated increased risk for transition to chronic pain among women compared to men, for conditions such as temporomandibular disorders, whiplash, postherpetic neuralgia, and chronic postoperative pain. For clinical studies (primarily postoperative pain), no sex differences in μ-opioid analgesia emerged overall. However, when restricting analyses to patient-controlled analgesia (PCA), women consumed lower amounts of μ-opioid medication, with the most significant effect developing for PCA morphine studies (a moderate effect size). Studies investigating μ-opioid analgesics tested against experimentally induced pain demonstrated greater morphine analgesia for women. This effect size was also moderate in magnitude. For mixed-action opioid agonist-antagonist medications (eg, butorphanol, nalbuphine, and pentazocine), women exhibit significantly higher analgesia than men in clinical studies, with a large effect size. It is now widely believed that pain affects men and women differently. While the sex hormones estrogen and testosterone certainly play a role in this phenomenon, psychology and culture, too, may account at least in part for differences in how men and women receive pain signals. For example, young children may learn to respond to pain based on how they are treated when they experience pain. Some children may be cuddled and comforted, while others may be encouraged to tough it out and to dismiss their pain. Many investigators are turning their attention to the study of gender differences and pain. Women, many experts now agree, recover more quickly from pain, seek help more quickly for their pain, and are less likely to allow pain to control their lives. They also are more likely to marshal a variety of resources-coping skills, support, and distraction-with which to deal with their pain. A review of the literature on gender and clinical pain reveals a disproportionate representation of women receiving treatment for many pain conditions and suggests that women report more severe pain, more frequent pain, and pain of longer duration than do men. Gender differences in pain perception have also been extensively studied in the laboratory, and ratings of experimentally induced pain also show some sex disparity, with females generally reporting lower pain thresholds and tolerance than males. However, there is little consensus on whether these apparent differences reflect the way men and women respond to pain, differing social rules for the expression of pain, or biologic differences in the way noxious stimuli are processed. The higher prevalence of chronic orofacial pain in women is a result of sex differences in generic pain mechanisms and of as-yet unidentified factors unique to the craniofacial system.

In 1992, an important publication by Karen Berkley highlighted the importance of sex-related issues in neuroscience research. This brief paper included a survey of 100 articles in reputable neuroscience journals, which found that 45% of the articles failed to report the sex of their subjects, and the author stated, "the differences between females and males, can and should be exploited in scientific research." Shortly thereafter, an editorial appeared in The Journal of Pain, which encouraged studying the differences between women and men, a topic that had been out of favor given the 1980s' emphasis on equality of the sexes. Women feel more pain than men, studies have shown. Women have more nerve receptors, which causes them to feel pain more intensely than men. On average, women have 34 nerve fibers per square centimeter of facial skin. Men average just 17. Earlier this year, separate research found that women report more pain throughout their lifetimes, in more areas of their bodies and for longer durations.

Women in pain are much more likely than men to receive prescriptions for sedatives, rather than pain medication, for their ailments. One study showed women who received coronary bypass surgery were only half as likely to be prescribed painkillers, as compared to men who had undergone the same procedure. These gender biases in our medical system can have serious and sometimes fatal repercussions. For instance, a 2000 study published in The New England Journal of Medicine found that women are seven times more likely than men to be misdiagnosed and discharged in the middle of having a heart attack. This occurred because the medical concepts of most diseases are based on understandings of male physiology, and women have altogether different symptoms than men when having a heart attack. Concerning chronic pain, 70% of the people it impacts are women. However, 80% of pain studies are conducted on male mice or human men. One of the few studies to research gender differences in the experience of pain found that women tend to feel it more of the time and more intensely than men. Biology and hormones are suspected of playing a role. Epidemiological evidence has clearly shown that pain is distributed differently in women and men. Overall, pain is reported more frequently by women than men, and specific pain conditions (e.g., migraine, fibromyalgia, irritable bowel syndrome, and temporomandibular disorders) are considerably more common in women than in men. We need to understand the underlying cause of these differences to fully understand how to treat patients better. If a clinician has developed his or her full view of pain based on the average man, anyone who responds differently to pain or analgesics than the average man seems unusual. Thus, we need to expand our expectations for what the "average" patient's pain experiences might be, because it varies wildly across people, and gender is one of the factors that seem to contribute to these differences.

Women have higher levels of estrogen and progesterone, and also are subject to more dramatic cyclic fluctuations in those and other hormones than men. It is clear that sex hormones are related to pain; however, this relationship is complicated. The link appears to be associated with the timing of the hormones, and for example, it might be estrogen withdrawal that precipitates pain rather than the average level of estrogen across the cycle. Also, while some evidence suggests that estrogens are associated with higher levels of pain, other studies have found that estrogens are associated with lower levels of pain. The organizational effects of sex hormones, the permanent impact of hormones in early development on the structure and function of our brains and bodies, also may play a role in sex differences in pain. Rodent models suggest that those first effects of hormones on pain can be even stronger than the impact of current hormone levels. In addition, research shows that other aspects of pain processing may vary between women and men. For example, evidence suggests that men show greater activation of μ-opioid receptors when subjected to pain compared to women. Brain imaging studies reveal some similarities, but also some differences between men and women in how the brain processes pain.

Furthermore, some evidence suggests that women have more densely innervated skin. Additionally, there are a variety of psychosocial contributors to pain. For example, women in the general population are more likely to have higher levels of depression and anxiety, both of which are known to potentially increase the risk of pain. Pain catastrophizing, magnification, rumination, and feeling of hopelessness are also typically higher in women than men. More upper pain catastrophizing scores have been found to correlate with higher pain intensity, pain-related disability, fear avoidance, and psychosocial distress. In contrast, women appear to have a broader repertoire of coping skills for pain, some of which are likely effective and some of which are characterized as being maladaptive. Stereotypic gender roles, masculinity, and femininity are correlated with pain as well. The extent to which gender roles are responsible for the sex difference in pain is hard to tell, but these roles may help explain why men tend to under-report pain or why women over-report pain, because of what is acceptable versus not acceptable according to gender roles. Male experimental animals injected with estrogen appear to have a lower tolerance for pain. Similarly, the presence of testosterone seems to elevate the tolerance for pain in female mice. Female mice deprived of estrogen during experiments react to stress similarly to male animals. Estrogen, therefore, may act as a sort of pain switch, turning on the ability to recognize pain. Kappa-opioids include the compounds nalbuphine (Nubain) and butorphanol (Stadol).

Research suggests that kappa-opioids provide better pain relief in women. Mu-opioids (morphine, oxycodone) offer better pain relief in men. Gendered norms about men and women with pain, present in research from different scientific fiends, illustrate prevailing hegemonic masculinity and and normativity in health care. The notion of gender is a construction and can be changed. Awareness about gendered norms and that they can lead to a consolidation of the dichotomous depiction of men and women is essential, both in research and clinical practice, to counteract gender bias in health care and to support health-care professionals in providing more equitable care.

The following "biological" factors contribute to a sex difference in pain. Gonadal hormonal influences on pain include both organizational and activation effects, which refer to long-term developmental impacts versus transient effects in adulthood, respectively. Clinical and experimental pain responses have been shown to vary across the menstrual cycle, with more significant clinical pain and pain sensitivity observed during the premenstrual and menstrual phases. Although, on average, these effects are modest in magnitude. Multiple "psychosocial" factors contribute to sex differences in pain. Gender roles, which are sculpted by both biology and social learning, have been associated with pain responses. In general, higher levels of masculinity and femininity are associated with lower and higher pain sensitivity, respectively. In general, women report higher levels of affective distress than men, including anxiety and depression, and both anxiety and depression are associated with increased risk of pain. Interestingly, several studies suggest that anxiety may be more strongly associated with pain among men than women. In contrast, among individuals with depression, women are more likely to report pain than men. Various biopsychosocial mechanisms contribute to sex differences in pain and analgesia. Recent years have witnessed substantially increased research regarding sex differences in pain. The expansive body of literature in this area clearly suggests that men and women differ in their responses to pain, with increased pain sensitivity and risk for clinical pain commonly being observed among women.

Differences in responsivity to pharmacological and non-pharmacological pain interventions have also been observed; however, these effects are not always consistent and appear dependent on treatment type and characteristics of both the pain and the provider. Although the specific etiological basis underlying these sex differences is unknown, it seems inevitable that multiple biological and psychosocial processes are contributing factors. For instance, emerging evidence suggests that genotype and endogenous opioid functioning play a causal role in these disparities, and considerable literature implicates sex hormones as factors influencing pain sensitivity. However, the specific modulatory effect of sex hormones on pain among men and women requires further exploration. Psychosocial processes such as pain coping and early-life exposure to stress may also explain sex differences in pain, in addition to stereotypical gender roles that may contribute to differences in pain expression. The future directions of this field of research are discussed with an emphasis aimed towards the further elucidation of mechanisms which may inform future efforts to develop sex-specific treatments. There is increasing evidence for sex differences in pain sensitivity and analgesic response. Clinical pain, both acute and chronic, and experimental pain models all show sex differences. While chronic pain is more common in women, the evidence on pain severity is less clear. Various psychosocial mechanisms may play a fundamental role in sex-related differences in pain. For instance, pain coping strategies have been found to differ between men and women. While men tend to use behavioral distraction and problem-focused tactics to manage pain, women tend to use a range of coping techniques including social support, positive self-statements, emotion-focused techniques, cognitive reinterpretation, and attentional focus. Multiple biopsychosocial mechanisms contribute to these sex differences in pain, including sex hormones, endogenous opioid function, genetic factors, pain coping and catastrophizing, and gender roles. At present, the available evidence does not support sex-specific tailoring of treatments; however, this is a likely outcome in the foreseeable future. Further research to elucidate the mechanisms driving sex differences in pain responses is needed in order to foster future interventions to reduce these disparities in pain. A study was done that aimed to examine whether or not there are gender differences in sweet stimulus-induced analgesia for cold pain in adults. In a randomized cross-over design, twenty men and 20 women held either a 24% sucrose solution or distilled water in their mouth before and while immersed their hand in cold water and their pain response was examined. Unlike the women, when the men held the sucrose solution in their mouth, the latency of the onset of pain significantly increased, compared with the distilled water. Meanwhile, the level of pain tolerance was not significantly different for both sexes. The findings reveal that the analgesic effect of a sweet stimulus on the pain threshold is influenced by gender differences in human adults, indicating that sweet stimulus-induced analgesia has a brief analgesic effect, particularly for men. Although more research is warranted, the sweet stimulus could be put to practical application as an adjunct to acute pain management for men.

References

J Integr Neurosci. 2011 Dec;10(4):537-45. MEG evaluation of taste by gender difference. Gemousakakis T[1], Kotini A, Anninos P, Zissimopoulos A, Prassopoulos P. Lab of Medical Physics, Department of Nuclear Physics, Medical School, Democritus University of Thrace, Alexandroupolis, 68100, Greece.

Berkley, Karen J (2009) Balancing nociception in cycling females. Pain 146:9-10

15. DIETARY HABITS

Dietary habits are fundamental issues to assess when modulating health and well-being; however, different nutritional panels may help individuals prevent acute and chronic pain. Many substances, known to be active antioxidants and anti-inflammatory compounds, should serve this fundamental task. Antinociceptive and analgesic natural compounds include flavonoids, terumbone from ginger root, curcuminoids, polyunsaturated fatty acids, and taurine. Recently, attention to the lifestyle of patients has been rapidly increasing in the field of pain therapy, particularly with regard to the role of nutrition in pain development and its management. Correct intake of trace elements and minerals is strategic to reduce inflammation-related pain. Osteoarthritis (OA) patients who are overweight or obese report higher levels of pain compared with their normal-weight OA counterparts. Evidence suggests that overweight or obese OA patients also experience pain relief from eating foods high in calories, fat or sugar. Eating to alleviate pain may be problematic because it can lead to additional weight gain, which may contribute to heightened pain.

A high-protein diet combined with restriction of carbohydrate and salt is recommended for patients with chronic pain. Protein contains the amino acids that are critical for many pain control functions, including formation of many neurotransmitters, hormones, muscle, and cartilage. Other components of a chronic pain diet ideally should contain select dietary supplements that help reduce inflammation, control weight, prevent osteopenia and osteoporosis, and regenerate nerve cells. Practitioners are urged to take a dietary history because the majority of chronic pain patients are woefully deficient in protein intake. Clearly, dietary counseling must be a component of chronic pain care. Plant-food supplements have anti-inflammatory effects. Fruits that are high in anthocyanins have shown to be anti- inflammatory. Carotenoids, found in red, yellow, and orange vegetables work via reducing pro-inflammatory pathways and causing a reduction in pain. Other vegetables, including broccoli, cauliflower, cabbage, and bok choy have various amount of a component that also reduces inflammatory pathways and reduce pain. Studies done on green tea extract show that a component in it has strong anti-inflammatory properties. Soy causes suppression of pro-inflammatory cytokines also. Both ginger and turmeric also work through multiple anti-inflammatory pathways and decrease pain.

Opioid treatment also has a profound effect on the endocrine–nutrition system, compounding the necessity of a pain diet. Patients on opioids commonly gain weight and prefer sweet foods. Weight gain may be profound, with some patients doubling their weight within a few years. Opioid use may cause blood sugar levels to be very unstable and may cause hypoglycemia. When the injury heals or the infection goes away, inflammation normally goes away too. However, sometimes your immune system gets turned on and stays on after the "crisis" has passed.   Over time, this can damage healthy cells and organs and cause constant pain in muscles, tissues, and joints. Chronic inflammation also can raise a patient's risk for heart disease, diabetes, certain cancers, and Alzheimer's disease. Opioids also cause a "sugar desire effect" on opioid receptors. Consequently, the combination of severe chronic pain and opioid treatment can cause deranged glucose metabolism in patients and a potent desire to ingest primarily sugars and starches, with little protein or fat intake. Some patients with pain give a history that about 2 hours after eating a carbohydrate load, such as a doughnut, bagel, or glass of fruit juice, their pain will flare. Obesity has been shown to have increased pro inflammatory cytokine levels. C-reactive protein specifically is directly related to amount of adipose tissue, which releases leptin to cause activation of the immune system and pro-inflammatory cytokines. A Western diet is one consisting of high intake of red meat, refined sugars, processed food, and saturated fats.

Vitamin D is known to decrease levels of inflammation. The chronic pain population, including those with fibromyalgia, is generally deficient in vitamin D. Pain patients without adequate vitamin D levels tend to stay on opioids twice as long and take twice as much of the drug as patients with appropriate vitamin

D levels. According to the Stanford University Medical School, the role of nutrition and its effect on pain is still in the early stages of research. There are several studies however that show certain substances in foods may help with reducing inflammation, improving mood and reducing the sensation of pain. Examples include: Omega-3 fatty acids. This is found in foods such as flaxseed, walnuts, halibut, shrimp and winter squash. Studies suggest that foods high in Omega-3 may reduce migraine headaches, inflammatory pain and pain associated with multiple sclerosis and arthritis. Tryptophan is present in dairy foods such as milk, yogurt, cottage and parmesan cheese, as well as other foods such as sesame, sunflower and pumpkin seeds. Chocolate, oats, bananas, poultry and turkey also have high levels of tryptophan. Tryptophan may be helpful in reducing neuropathic pain and improving sleep. Furthermore, foods high in fiber are effective in preventing constipation which is known to aggravate back pain. Soy-enriched diets may have positive effects in reducing neuropathic pain. Green tea and cherries may also have pain-relieving properties as well.

The evidence for dietary modification to improve chronic pain is immense. Diet and nutritional supplements are important factors in inflammation and pain, and modification of diet in patients with chronic pain should be a part of a comprehensive treatment plan. Obesity is a risk factor for chronic pain, and obese patients have a higher prevalence of chronic pain. Obesity, deficient nutrient intake, and poor eating behavior are highly prevalent in patients with chronic pain on long-term opioid therapy. Patients may be surprised to learn that an individual can help minimize pain through one's food choices. Eating gluten can cause generalized pain. Many people have a sensitivity to gluten in which the body recognizes gluten as a foreign pathogen and releases inflammatory chemicals. An inflammatory response can be very painful, and if a patient is gluten intolerant but ingests gluten on a regular basis, that patient may have chronic inflammation causing widespread pain.

Gluten is a protein found in wheat, rye, barley, and some processed oats. It is also in many processed foods. Egg yolks contain arachidonic acid, which studies have shown is one of the main fatty acids involved in inflammation. Diets high in arachidonic acid may lead to a constant level of inflammation, and thus, pain. Red meat can contribute to chronic pain in a few ways. First, meat is high in purines. When a person ingests dietary purines, the body breaks them down into uric acid, which can cause the excruciatingly painful condition known as gout. Likewise, meat is also high in fats containing arachidonic acid, which can cause inflammation and pain. Many foods are fried in oils high in omega-6 fatty acids. The body needs a balance of omega-3 and omega-6 fatty acids. The omega-3 to omega-6 ratio should be 1:1; however, in the typical Western diet it is about 1:15. Omega-6 fats at this high of a level in the human body are pro-inflammatory, which can lead to inflammation and chronic pain. Processed foods are foods those which come in a bag, box, package, or can and may cause chronic pain and inflammation for a number of reasons. Some of the pain causing ingredients in processed foods include gluten, trans fats, high levels of omega-6 fatty acids, and artificial chemicals.

Some foods on the other hand may relieve pain. Dark leafy greens such as spinach, kale, and Swiss chard are high in antioxidants and nutrients that fight oxidative stress. Eating greens can also help prevent osteoporosis. Raw walnuts are high in omega-3 fats, which can help to balance the omega-3 vs omega-6 ratio, which decreases inflammatory pain. Avocados are high in vitamin K and vitamin K can reduces arthritic pain. Sea Vegetables: like kelp and dulse contain fucoidans which are polysaccharides that studies have shown to reduce pain. Sea vegetables are also good for providing many trace minerals, as well as B vitamins and iron. Acai berries are high in antioxidants and omega-3 fatty acids, both of which are powerful anti-inflammatory substances. Antioxidants fight free radicals, which can damage cells and cause pain, while omega-3 fats fight inflammation. ginger decreased muscle pain by 25 percent. Ginger may be effective at relieving the pain of osteoarthritis. Tart cherry juice is high in antioxidants and may relieve the pain of osteoarthritis. Turmeric may also be effective for relieving the pain of osteoarthritis. Flaxseeds are also high in omega-3 fatty acids. Eating foods high in omega-3 fatty acids can reduce inflammation, and pain.

The evidence for dietary modification to improve chronic pain is vast and continues to grow. Diet and nutritional supplements are nociceptive known to be important factors in decreasing inflammation and chronic pain, and modification of the diet in patients with chronic pain should be a part of a comprehensive pain treatment plan. Many serious inflammatory disorders and nutrient deficiencies induce chronic pain, and anti-inflammatory diets have been applied successfully to modify the inflammatory symptoms causing chronic pain. Numerous scientific data and clinical investigations have demonstrated that long-term inflammation could lead to an inappropriate or exaggerated sensibility to pain. Also, some non-steroidal anti-inflammatory drugs (NSAID), which directly act on the many enzymes involved in pain and inflammation, including cyclooxygenases, are used to dampen the algesic signal to the central nervous system, reducing the responses of soft C-fibers to pain stimuli. On the other hand, there are a few reports from both health authorities and physicians, reporting that decreased transmission of pain signals can be achieved and improved, depending on the patient's dietary habit. Many nutrients, as well as a suitable level of exercise (resistance training), is the best method for improving the total mitochondrial capacity in muscle cells, which can lead to a reduction in sensitivity to pain, particularly by lowering the inflammatory signaling to C-fibers. According to the current literature, it could be proposed that chronic pain results from the changed ratio of neuropeptides, hormones, and poor nutritional status, often related to an underlying inflammatory disorder.

Nutritional interventions can have a positive effect on the pain experience through the indirect inhibitory effect on prostaglandin E2 and attenuation of mitochondrial dysfunction caused by ischemia/reperfusion in skeletal muscle, improving the intracellular antioxidant defense system. These data highlight the need for more nutrition studies where chronic pain is the primary outcome, using accurate interventions. To date, no nutritional recommendation for chronic pain has been officially proposed.

Food provides the building blocks for a strong, healthy and energetic body. However, eating the wrong foods increases one's risk of developing heart disease and cancer, but one's diet also contributes to increased pain sensitivity. Pain sensation is transmitted by nerve cells that travel to and from the brain. The sensitivity of these nerve cells affects the way that people process pain. If these nerve cells are overly sensitive, one may experience exaggerated pain compared what might be normal for other people. Certain foods trigger the release of chemicals that increase this nerve sensitivity. Vegetables in the nightshade family release a chemical that in some people aggravates the pain and stiffness associated with arthritis. Foods in this family include tomatoes, potatoes, and eggplant. Potato chips are especially troublesome because they are deep fried in omega-6 oils that are highly inflammatory and also contribute to increased pain and inflammation.

Foods containing yeast and gluten can increase pain sensitivity as well. Yeast is most commonly found in breads and baked goods and it contributes to the growth of fungus. Fungus is a stressor on the body and increases pain sensitivity. Gluten is a small protein found in anything made with wheat, rye, or barley. This protein binds to tissues throughout the body and can cause increased pain sensitivity. Dairy contains two proteins that cause an immune response in the body: whey and casein. Sensitivity to these proteins results in pain and inflammation. Dairy products also contain a type of saturated fat which the body uses to produce a chemical that stimulates pain sensation. Less consumption of this type of fat results in reduced signaling of pain. The reason inflammation is so critical is that it has been found to be a player in almost every chronic disease. Here are laboratory indications that someone may have a chronic inflammatory condition: white blood cell count, sedimentation rate (ESR), and the high sensitivity C-reactive protein (hs CRP).

Certain foods trigger the release of chemicals that increase pain nerve sensitivity in one's. body. Vegetables in the nightshade family release a chemical that in some people aggravates the pain and stiffness associated with arthritis. Foods in this family include tomatoes, potatoes, and eggplant. Potato chips are especially troublesome because they are deep fried in omega-6 oils that are highly inflammatory and also contribute to increased pain and inflammation. Foods containing yeast and gluten can increase the pain sensitivity as well. Gluten is a small protein found in anything made with wheat, rye, or barley. This protein binds to tissues throughout the body and can cause a variety of problems from headaches and sinus trouble to digestive issues and increased pain sensitivity. Dairy products also contain a type of saturated fat which the body uses to produce a chemical that stimulates pain sensation. Less consumption of this type of fat results in reduced signaling of pain. Products containing aspartame (Nutrasweet, Equal) have also been associated with pain, numbness, tingling, and muscle and joint pain. Aspartame activates nerve cells that increase pain sensitivity.

Reference

Curr Med Chem. 2019 Jul 12. doi:
10.2174/0929867326666190712172015. [Epub ahead of print]
Insights on nutrients as analgesics in chronic pain. Bjørklund
G, Chirumbolo S, Dadar M, Pen JJ, Doşa MD, Pivina
L, Semenova Y, Aaseth J.

16. CAN A DIET DECREASE PAIN?

Research shows that diet should be an integral part of a pain management program. Patients with chronic pain need a high-protein-intake diet, with avoidance of carbohydrate-induced episodes of hypoglycemia and weight gain. Considerable scientific information and clinical observation have accumulated in recent years that chronic pain, particularly the debilitating, severe form that requires opioid treatment, needs a chronic pain diet. The fundamental principle of the diet is that patients with chronic pain need a high protein diet with avoidance of carbohydrates. It is also is intended to promote strength, movement, energy, and mental function. The dietary supplements also recommended are intended to assist regeneration of tissue and prevent osteopenia and osteoporosis.

Opioid treatment has a profound effect on the endocrine–nutrition system, compounding the necessity of a pain diet. Weight gain may be profound, with some patients doubling their weight within a few years. Opioid use may cause blood sugar levels to be very unstable and may cause hypoglycemia. Opioids cause a "sugar desire effect" on opioid receptors. Consequently, the combination of severe chronic pain and opioid treatment can cause changes of glucose metabolism in patients and a desire to ingest primarily sugars and starches, with little protein or fat intake. Clinical observations of patients with chronic pain who require opioid treatment support the scientific research and the adverse effects of pain and opioids on the endocrine–nutrition systems. Pain patients with chronic pain report a gross deficiency of protein intake. It is recommended that pain practitioners take a dietary history for protein intake and examine the patient for muscle loss and weakness. Patients with pain may drink large amounts of sugar drinks and milk. A major element of the diet recommended here is stabilization of blood sugars.

A chronic pain diet should be based on high-protein intake. Endogenous pain relievers are protein derivatives. Amino acids enter the blood from the intestine and travel to locations in the liver, glands, and brain, where they are building blocks for compounds critical to pain relief. These include endorphin, dopamine, serotonin, and γ-aminobutyric acid (GABA). Insulin and thyroid hormones are derived from amino acids. The complaint of weakness by patients with severe pain may have many causes, but a lack of protein is one of them. Furthermore, the receptors to which pain-modulating neurotransmitters (endorphin, serotonin, and GABA) attach are protein moieties. A number of amino acids are required to build muscle. The amino acid proline is the major building block of collagen, which is essential for the development of cartilage and intervertebral discs.

Glucagon is secreted by the liver in response to protein ingestion. Glucagon increases blood glucose levels, and blocks glucose storage as fat. Eating protein with every meal and every time sugar and starches are eaten will prevent a rapid rise in insulin, storage of any excess glucose as fat, and hypoglycemia that results in carbohydrate cravings and possible pain flares. On the other hand, many foods that contain protein, such as fish and green vegetables, contain anti-inflammatory agents. The major dietary recommendation for patients with chronic pain is to eat protein foods with each meal and to not eat or drink carbohydrates. It is well known that caffeine raises brain dopamine levels, which gives a little extra pain relief. High cholesterol, lipids, and glucose are almost universal in patients with uncontrolled pain because of excess cortisol secretion from the adrenal gland. Good pain control will usually lower high serum lipid and glucose levels. Adequate intake of protein with carbohydrate restriction also will help to control lipid and glucose levels. Many patients with pain have pain sites in the spine, hips, knees, and feet that may be aggravated by excess weight. A medication that will relieve pain may suppress the body's metabolism and cause weight gain. There are many amino acid powders, bars, and drinks marketed to athletes and bodybuilders. They make excellent supplements for patients with chronic pain. A high-protein diet combined with restriction of carbohydrate and salt is recommended for patients with chronic pain. Protein contains the amino acids that are critical for many pain control functions, including formation of many neurotransmitters, hormones, muscle, and cartilage. Other components of a chronic pain diet ideally should contain select dietary supplements that help reduce inflammation, control weight, prevent osteopenia and osteoporosis, and regenerate nerve cells. A consultation with a dietician is highly recommended for patients suffering from chronic pain.

References

Mysels DJ, Vosburg SK, Bengci I, Levin FR, Sullivan MA. Course of weight change during naltrexone versus methadone maintenance for opioid-dependent patients. J Opioid Manag. 2011;7(1):47-53.

Tennant FS, Herman L. Normalization of serum cortisol concentration with opioid treatment of severe chronic pain. Pain Med. 2002;3(2):132-134.

17. MICHELLE OBAMA

In 2009, First Lady Michelle Obama planted the White House Kitchen Garden on the South Lawn to initiate a national conversation around the health and wellbeing of our nation. That conversation led to Let's Move! an initiative launched in 2010 dedicated to helping children and families lead healthier lives.

At the start of Let's Move!, President Obama established the first-ever Task Force on Childhood Obesity to develop a national action plan to mobilize the public and private sectors and engage families and communities in an effort to improve the health of our children. Combining comprehensive strategies with common sense, Let's Move! is about putting children on the path to a healthy future during their earliest months and years; giving parents helpful information and fostering environments that support healthy choices; providing healthier foods in our schools; ensuring that every family has access to healthy, affordable food; and helping children become more physically active.

First lady Michelle Obama subsequently unveiled the new food label in 2013, which represented major victories both for her legacy and the efforts of advocacy groups and prominent scientists who have argued that the previous version made it difficult for consumers to assess the nutritional quality of any given food item. This change made a real difference in providing families across the country the information they need to make healthy choices. The change addressed some of the early arguments waged by the sugar industry, which argued that having a line that says "sugars" and another that says "added sugars" would be confusing, since it wouldn't make clear that the latter is part of the first. The FDA addressed that problem by changing "sugars" to "total sugars" and adding "includes" to the "added sugars" line. Among the many changes, which included larger type for the number of calories and servings per container, is a new line located just beneath "total sugars." It tells consumers exactly how much of the sugar was added by the manufacturer, and what percentage of the daily recommended intake that added sugar comprises.

The sugar industry however used its political influence and large sums of cash to defend its place in the American diet. Documents revealed how the industry skewed the government's medical research in the 1960s on the role sugar played in tooth decay and ultimately, how much sugar officials recommended for the American diet. The American Beverage Association, which represents prominent purveyors of sugary drinks, such as Coca-Cola and Pepsi, spent millions of dollars battling various soda tax bills that have popped up in recent years. The result had been a series of victories that have helped infuse what we eat with a great deal more sugar than virtually any doctor would recommend. Sugar is so prevalent in the American diet that it creeps into the strangest things, including Clamato juice, Subway sandwiches, Luna granola bars, Yoplait yogurt and California Pizza Kitchen salads, etc. The average American consumes more than 126 grams of sugar per day, which is slightly more than three 12-ounce cans of Coca-Cola and more than twice the average sugar intake of 54 countries observed by Euromonitor, including Canada and Britain.

The hope was that the new label, which makes clear when a food manufacturer has relied heavily on sugar to make its product tasty, will help Americans make more informed choices about the foods they eat. The daily recommended limit is 50 grams of added sugar, which means that a can of soda will look much less appealing to anyone who bothers to glance at the label. A regular Pepsi, for example, has 69 grams of sugar, so it would have to be listed has having 138 percent of the Daily Value for added sugars. This is precisely the sort of information an industry whose bottom line is directly tied to the decadent use of sugar could do without. Childhood obesity rates are indeed showing small declines for the first time in decades, especially in cities with aggressive nutrition policies. As Mrs. Obama pointed out, "Let's Move" has helped call attention to the childhood obesity crisis, and one of her cornerstone achievements was comprehensive school lunch reform that increased funding for public school meals and gave the USDA the ability to regulate foods sold in schools.

Besides school lunch reform, however, "Let's Move" has deliberately veered away from pushing actual legislation, instead focusing on personal responsibility in nutrition and fitness. That's a very different approach than the one Mrs. Obama took during the inception of her fight against childhood obesity. In 2010, the First Lady gave a fiery speech at a Grocery Manufacturers Association conference, arguing that changing personal habits won't work if big companies like Kraft and General Mills continue to target children with misleading ads for sugary, fatty food.

While self-regulating companies can make a big difference, their standards tend to be far more lenient than federal regulations. In 2011, a federal task force drafted voluntary guidelines for marketing food to children only to see them killed by a lobbying blitz by Walt Disney, Nestlé, Kellogg and General Mills which were all companies involved in Let's Move partnerships. Meanwhile, "Let's Move" stayed silent on the proposed standards, despite Mrs. Obama's earlier condemnation of junk food advertising. A few months later, the First Lady announced a separate agreement with Disney with significantly watered-down guidelines to end marketing junk food to kids. This avoidance of policy change may have had something to do with the food lobby's influence in Obama's White House. According to a Reuters analysis, 50 food and beverage groups have spent more than $175 million in lobbying since Obama took office, dwarfing the $83 million spent in the last 3 years of the Bush administration.

After sustained lobbying from the packaged food and beverage industry, the Food and Drug Administration announced an indefinite delay in the launch of Nutrition Fact labels that were intended to help Americans eat more healthfully. The labels, championed by former first lady Michelle Obama, were supposed to add a special line for "added sugars" and emphasize calorie content in large, bold text. They had been scheduled for rollout in July 2018, with a one-year extension for smaller manufacturers. The delay was the latest reversal of the Obama administration's nutrition reforms under President Trump. On April 27, the FDA also delayed rules that would have required calorie counts on restaurant menus. A week later, the Department of Agriculture loosened the minimum requirements for the amount of whole grain in school lunches and delayed future sodium reductions.

A new Nutrition Facts label that highlights the amount of added sugars in food could prevent nearly 1 million cases of heart disease and type 2 diabetes, a new study suggested. The new label, first proposed by the U.S. Food and Drug Administration in May 2016, adds a new line under the Total Carbohydrate category that details the amount of sugar that has been added on top of the sugars already contained in a food product. If consumers had access to this new label, their food choices could prevent more than 350,000 cases of heart disease and nearly 600,000 cases of type 2 diabetes over the next two decades, researchers predicted using a computer model. When

Donald Trump took office in January and then appointed Sonny Perdue as USDA secretary, many in "big food" sighed in relief. After all, neither man is known for supporting healthier diets or stricter food regulations. In fact, in the first few months of the Trump presidency, we saw the Obama-led changes to school lunch programs rolled back to eliminate the lower sodium and whole grains regulations and chocolate-flavored milk with added sugar put back on menus. Earlier this month, we witnessed the poultry industry's lobbying to allow for faster speeds for inspection lines; historical data has shown that faster speeds lead to both food safety issues and worker injuries and illnesses.

"In North America, we are undergoing one of the world's most serious obesity epidemics, mainly due to the consumption of unhealthy food and beverages," said Alejandro Calvillo, Executive Director, El Poder del Consumidor, and member of the Nutritional Health Alliance in Mexico. "Consumers urgently need access to clear information and warnings about these products. A trade agreement should not defy the population's rights to information and to health in the face of this dire health problem in our region."

The Grocery Manufacturers Association (GMA) and other food industry groups had asked for an extension to 2021. The new nutrition label would allow consumers to have a better and clearer idea of the amounts of certain nutrients in their foods, as well as of ingredients they might choose to reduce or avoid, such as added sugars. intake due to kidney issues, or medication interactions which is information that was not on the old label. This final guidance, "Declaration of Added Sugars on Honey, Maple Syrup, and Certain Cranberry Products," provides clarification for companies that produce single-ingredient sugars and syrups, in addition to those who produce cranberry products. Single-ingredient sugars are intended to be consumed alone or added to foods by consumers, and thus will be an added sugar to the diet when consumed. As companies who produce these products began to look at how they would implement the new label, they raised concerns about how consumers would perceive the Added Sugars declaration on their product labels. Additionally, the Agriculture Improvement Act of 2018, commonly referred to as the "Farm Bill," stated that Nutrition Facts labels cannot require the declaration of the gram amount of Added Sugars for single-ingredient sugars, honey, agave and syrups, including maple syrup.

After reviewing and considering the comments made to the February 2018 draft guidance, as well as fulfilling the legislative requirement in the 2018 Farm Bill, legislators were finalizing this guidance in a way that provides consumers with information as to how consumption of these products can be accommodated within the recommendations of the dietary guidelines, while at the same time reducing the potential for consumers to misinterpret single-ingredient sugars and syrups as having additional sugars added to them.

The final guidance issued recently explains that for single-ingredient sugars, the Nutrition Facts label will still include a line for Total Sugars with the amount per serving expressed in grams; however, the line below it which has been reserved for Added Sugars will only provide a percent Daily Value for Added Sugars. We are exercising enforcement discretion to allow for the use of a "†" symbol immediately following the percent Daily Value declaration for Added Sugars, which leads consumers to a statement that provides information about the gram amount of Added Sugars, as well as information about how that amount of sugar contributes to the percent Daily Value. As an example, for a single-ingredient sugar that provides 10 grams of sugar per serving, manufacturers are encouraged to include a "†" symbol after the percent Daily Value declaration for Added Sugars that refers the consumer to information that reads: 'One serving adds 10g of sugar to your diet and represents 20% of the Daily Value for Added Sugars.' The goal with this final guidance is to help consumers understand that these single-ingredient sugars have no additional sugars added to them, while also conveying how their consumption will contribute to the amount of Added Sugars consumed in a day.

Additionally, the final guidance provides information related to the labeling of added sugars on certain cranberry products. Since cranberries are naturally tart and contain very little natural sugar, the manufacturers of these products frequently add sugar to make them more palatable. The makers of these products have stated that even after adding sugar, their products typically have the equivalent total sugar content of other fruit products that do not have sugars added. Therefore, in instances where sugar is added and it does not exceed the level in a comparable fruit product, such as cranberry juice cocktail as compared to unsweetened grape juice, we are stating our intent to exercise enforcement discretion to allow the Nutrition Facts label to include a symbol that leads the consumer to a statement outside the Nutrition Facts label indicating that sugar has been added because cranberries are naturally tart. The statement can also indicate that *the* 2015-2020 Dietary Guidelines for Americans includes language that there is room for limited amounts of added sugars in the diet, including from nutrient-dense foods like naturally tart fruit. Alternatively, the statement could refer to the 2015-2020 Dietary Guidelines for Americans recommended limit for added sugars of no more than 10% of calories. The intent with this additional information is to help American consumers more easily understand how certain sweetened cranberry products part of a healthy dietary pattern can be.

In implementing this final guidance today, the government has made sure to allow ample time for manufacturers to comply. Therefore, this guidance states the intent to exercise enforcement discretion so that any single-ingredient sugar or cranberry product that is impacted by this guidance will have until July 1, 2021 to switch to the new label. The government want to ensure that manufacturers have time to redesign their packaging and adhere to the new labeling requirements.

In updating the Nutrition Facts label and later releasing the Nutrition Innovation Strategy, the goal has been to provide consumers with the information they need to make informed decisions about their diet and health, including with the products they are eating every day. Other changes that consumers are seeing on the new label include adjusted serving sizes so that the amounts of calories and nutrients listed on the label more accurately reflect what is customarily consumed. Additionally, Americans are seeing a change in which nutrients are declared, as vitamin D and potassium are now required on the label because Americans do not always get the recommended amounts.

The Added Sugars declaration is one more piece of information that consumers can use to make informed decisions about their diet. The goal in issuing this final guidance is to help consumers better understand how consumption of single-ingredient sugars and certain cranberry products can be accommodated within recommended limits for added sugars in healthy diets.

When the US, Canada, and Mexico inked NAFTA in 1994, the American sugar industry was able negotiate a deal that put a limit on the amount of sugar Mexico could import from the US for 14 years. In 2008, when that limit expired, Mexico gained autonomous access to the US sugar market. Per the agreement, no more than 53% of Mexican sugar exported into the US could be refined. The remaining 47% from Mexico had to be raw, allowing US sugar processors to refine it themselves. American sugar processors have long complained that Mexico has exported a type of sugar that is technically raw but in practice needs so little processing that it can be used as if it were already refined. That has hurt the American sugar processing business, and the industry lashed out at Mexico by filing a complaint in 2014 with the US Department of Commerce accusing the Mexican sugar industry of unfair trading practices.
The department sided with US companies, and prepared to assess the possibility of encumbering Mexico with punitive duties on the sugar it sends into the US.

The Obama administration dismissed the case, so now the decision landed on Trump's commerce secretary, Wilbur Ross, who faces the unenviable task of trying to strike a compromise or risk igniting a trade war with one of America's most important trade partners. One of the demands processors have sought is a tweak to the ratio of sugar Mexico can ship into the US. They are asking that from now on, 85% of Mexican sugar must be raw, and 15% refined. Mexican authorities have countered that such demands are proof the US sugar industry is attempting to eliminate competition with Mexican refined sugar. If a compromise cannot be met and the US decides to impose duties on US sugar, it would send a ripple effect throughout the food industry. A group of Congressional lawmakers sent a letter to the US Department of Commerce, asking Ross to do everything he can to avoid placing tariffs on Mexico. "An increase in the tariffs on imported sugar would increase the price of food to American consumers."

Meanwhile, major food manufacturing companies and the corn syrup industry say erecting a tariff on Mexican sugar would wind up hurting US jobs and make food more costly for Americans. Those companies are worried because, if the US did raise tariffs, Mexico could easily retaliate by limiting the amount of high-fructose corn syrup, a sugar substitute, it imports from the US. That's not good news for American corn or corn syrup producers, who've sold more than $3 billion in sweetener to Mexico over the last five years. Any deal the two countries wind up striking could further shake up the politically volatile situation in the US. Trump, who garnered the overwhelming support of the agriculture sector during his presidential campaign, could also risk be alienating that important part of his base if tariffs are raised. This group includes the powerful corn growers, who have a stake in the sugar battle as corn is an integral component of high-fructose corn syrup, a sugar substitute.

In Nebraska, for instance, the state corn board, the US Grains Council, and the National Corn Growers Association, have mobilized to organize town hall meetings and arrange transportation for farmers. These farmers have one main goal: to get lawmakers to support NAFTA, according to state media. Mexico is Nebraska's biggest export market for corn, making up close to $290 million of the state's economy. Trump's threat to shake up trade pacts should come as no surprise, of course, as he promised to renegotiate or terminate NAFTA on the campaign trail. Considering the income made and the politics in the sugar, industry one cannot expect that the medical establishment will interfere with the sugar industry itself. As a result, individual medical practitioners and medical societies will themselves have to warn their patients about the dangers of sugar on an individual's health.

18. PAIN OVERVIEW

Dr. Ackerman has built his career educating patients, other physicians, medical students and residents and fellows about the highest standards in medical practice. He is a strong proponent of ethics in medicine and the accuracy of medical information which inspired him to write this book on the effects of nutrition on pain management.

Medical professionals and researchers are trying to determine the best ways to impede and treat chronic pain. If a patient's pain is due to inflammation, what and how much the patient eats is an important piece of the problem. Many conditions are associated with inflammation, including injury or infection, rheumatoid arthritis, inflammatory bowel disease, pelvic inflammatory disorder, Crohn's disease, colitis, atherosclerosis, diabetes, hepatitis, asthma, chronic obstructive pulmonary disease, vasculitis, autoimmune disorders, some cancers, sinusitis, and chronic periodontitis. While some types of pain can only be relieved by medical treatments, chronic pain due to inflammation can be improved by following a healthier diet. A reasonably healthy diet allows a body to better manage pain.

With back pain, joint pain, or any type of musculoskeletal pain, it hurts to pick up and carry something heavy. For the same reason, when a patient is overweight this individual is carrying extra pounds that are putting excess weight on the muscles, bones, and joints which causes pain. Any existing pain from disease or damage to a body can only worsen with added weight. Studies suggest that people who carry excess fat, particularly in the abdominal area, are at higher risk of developing low-grade inflammation throughout their bodies. That extra body fat plays a role in painful health problems such as fibromyalgia, chronic headaches, abdominal pain, pelvic pain, arthritis, and lower back pain.

Eating a high-fat diet activates cells that promote inflammation in your body's fatty tissue. That inflammation contributes to obesity and medical conditions associated with being overweight, including insulin resistance, diabetes, and heart disease. Red meat particularly processed red meat like cold cuts, sausages, and bacon is high in saturated fat and, when regularly consumed as part of a traditional American diet, has been linked to low-grade chronic inflammation as well as pain.

Many of the studies linking omega-3 fatty acids consumed from fatty fish like salmon and herring, fish oils, flaxseeds, and other sources to the reduction of inflammation and chronic pain have involved patients with arthritis and cardiovascular heart disease. At least one study also found that even when inflammation was controlled by medication, omega-3s helped reduce residual pain that was due to factors other than inflammation. These findings led researchers to conclude that omega-3 fatty acids may be beneficial in the early stages of rheumatoid arthritis, before inflammation intensifies. However, not all fatty acids are created equal and the ratio of omega-3 fatty acids to omega-6 fatty acids (from palm, soybean, rapeseed, and sunflower) also matters. A study of people with knee osteoarthritis whose diet was higher in omega-6 fats than omega-3 fats had more pain and more physical limitations than those who had a higher ratio of omega-3 fats to omega 6. This supports the theory that the balance of different fats in one's diet from different sources is as important as the types and amount of fat a person eats.

Eating a plant-based diet may hold the key to fighting inflammation, obesity, and conditions that lead to painful chronic disease. A traditional Mediterranean-style diet, when used to replace a traditional American diet, has been shown to reduce markers of chronic inflammation as well as lowering the risk of developing or dying from chronic diseases associated with inflammation. To help reduce inflammation, one should increase fiber in the diet, and improve one's overall health, and substitute high-protein plant foods such as legumes, nuts, and whole grains for some or all of the meat in the daily diet.

For centuries, practitioners of Chinese herbal medicine, Ayurvedic medicine, and other alternative and complementary forms of health care have long known the value of medical herbs and spices, including those that reduce pain and inflammation. More recently, scientists have confirmed the anti-inflammatory effects of herbs and spices such as turmeric, cinnamon, ginger, cayenne, sage, and rosemary and continue to study their role in fighting pain. For instance, compounds in ginger are particularly effective in the gastro-intestinal tract. Cinnamon has been shown to reduce the severity and duration of menstrual pain. Turmeric can reduce joint pain in rheumatoid arthritis, inhibit cancer cells, and slow the progression of diabetes-related disorders.

Substances in rosemary have the potential to fight a variety of inflammatory diseases, bronchial asthma, peptic ulcer, and liver toxicity, and protect against cancer. Some dietary changes may not be appropriate for some medical conditions. In order to get a sense of what is best for a patient, the patient should speak with a doctor or a registered dietitian before making any drastic changes. And since nutrients, herbs, and other substances in supplemental form can sometimes interfere with medical treatments, or cause problems of their own, it is also important for a patient to tell his/her health care provider what vitamins or supplements he or she is taking.

References

Lee CG, Lee JK, Kang Y-S, et al. Visceral abdominal obesity is associated with an increased risk of irritable bowel syndrome. The American Journal of Gastroenterology. 2015; 110:310-319.

Collins B, Hoffman J, Martinez K, et al. A polyphenol-rich fraction obtained from table grapes decreases adiposity, insulin resistance and markers of inflammation and impacts gut microbiota in high-fat-fed mice. The Journal of Nutritional Biochemistry. 2016; 31:150-165.

Okifuji A, Hare BD. The association between chronic pain and obesity. Journal of Pain Research. 2015; 8:399-408.

19. SUGAR BEHAVIOR

The link between sugar and addictive behavior is tied to the fact that, when a person eats sugar, opioids and dopamine are released. When a certain behavior causes an excess release of dopamine, one feels a pleasurable "high" that people are inclined to re-experience, and so repeat the behavior.   In medicine physicians use 'addiction' to describe a tragic situation where someone's brain chemistry has been altered to compel them to repeat a substance or activity despite harmful consequences. Evidence is mounting that too much added sugar could lead to true addiction as well. The link between sugar and addictive behavior is tied to the fact that, when a person eats sugar, opioids and dopamine are released. Dopamine is a neurotransmitter that is a key part of the "reward circuit" associated with addictive behavior.

When a certain behavior causes an excess release of dopamine, you feel a pleasurable "high" that persons are inclined to re-experience, and so repeat the behavior. As one repeats that behavior more and more, the brain adjusts to release less dopamine. The only way to feel the same "high" as before is to repeat the behavior in increasing amounts and frequency. This is known as substance abuse. Research shows that sugar can be even more addicting than cocaine. Sugar activates the opiate receptors in the brain and affects the reward center, which leads to compulsive behavior, despite the negative consequences like weight gain, headaches, hormone imbalances, and more. Studies suggest that every time a person eats sweets, they are reinforcing those neuropathways, causing the brain to become increasingly hardwired to crave sugar, building up a tolerance like any other drug," she adds.

Research on rats from Connecticut College has shown that Oreo cookies activate more neurons in the brain's pleasure center than cocaine does (and just like humans, the rats would eat the filling first). And a 2008 Princeton study found that, under certain circumstances, not only could rats become dependent on sugar, but this dependency correlated with several aspects of addiction, including craving, binging, and withdrawal. Researchers believe that the casual link between sugar and illegal drugs doesn't just make for dramatic headlines. Not only is there truth to it, but they determined the rewards experienced by the brain after consuming sugar are even "more rewarding and attractive" than the effects of cocaine. Medical addiction changes brain chemistry to cause binging, craving, withdrawal symptoms, and sensitization." "Excess added sugar can do this too, through changes in the same pathways as addiction to amphetamines or alcohol. Sugar addiction could be an even harder habit to break, according to recent evidence about how added sugar affects our stress hormones." Sugar is also much more prevalent, available, and socially acceptable than amphetamines or alcohol, and so harder to avoid. But whether or not sugar is more addictive than

cocaine, researchers and nutritionists are in agreement that
sugar has addictive properties, and people need to be getting
less of it. There is an increasing body of research demonstrating
that sugar can stimulate the brain's reward processing center in a
manner that mimics what we see with some recreational drugs.
In certain individuals with certain predispositions, this could
manifest as an addiction to sugary foods."

The World Health Organization (WHO) cautions people to
reduce their intake of "free sugars" to less than 10 percent of
daily calories since 1989, saying that doing so can lower the
risk for being obese, overweight, or experiencing tooth decay.
"Free sugars" include both the sugars naturally found in honey
and fruit juice, and sugar added to food and drinks. On food
labels, added sugars include words such as glucose, corn syrup,
brown sugar, dextrose, maltose, and sucrose, as well as many
others. In 2015, they further suggested reducing free sugar
intake to less than 5 percent of calories, about 6 teaspoons. In
the United States, sugars account for 14 percent of the average
person's calorie intake. Most of this comes from beverages,
including energy drinks, alcoholic drinks, soda, fruit drinks, and
sweetened coffee and teas. Other common sources are snacks.
These don't just include obvious perpetrators, like brownies,
cookies, doughnuts, and ice cream. A person can also find large
quantities of added sugar in bread, salad dressing, granola bars,
and even fat-free yogurt. High-calorie sweeteners are in over

95 percent of granola bars, cereals, and sugar-sweetened beverages, most often in the form of corn syrup, sorghum, and cane sugar.

The ODPHP 2015-2020 Dietary Guidelines suggest cutting consumption of added sugars to less than 10 percent of calories per day. To help consumers, the Food and Drug Administration has developed a new food label source that lists added sugars separately, which manufacturers were required to use beginning in 2018. Reducing sugar, especially concentrated sugars, not only limits the amount of sugars ingested but also makes less sweet foods seem sweeter. Dopamine is a neurotransmitter that is a key part of the "reward circuit" associated with addictive behavior. When a certain behavior causes an excess release of dopamine, that individual may feel a pleasurable "high" that he/she are inclined to re-experience, and so repeat the behavior. As one repeats that behavior more and more, the brain adjusts to release less dopamine. The only way to feel the same "high" as before is to repeat the behavior in increasing amounts and frequency. This is known as substance abuse.

"Research shows that sugar can be even more addicting than cocaine," says Cassie Bjork, R.D., L.D., founder of Healthy Simple Life. "Sugar activates the opiate receptors in our brain and affects the reward center, which leads to compulsive behavior, despite the negative consequences like weight gain, headaches, hormone imbalances, and more." "Studies suggest that every time we eat sweets, we are reinforcing those neuropathways, causing the brain to become increasingly hardwired to crave sugar, building up a tolerance like any other drug," she adds.

Research on rats from Connecticut College has shown that Oreo cookies activate more neurons in the brain's pleasure center than cocaine does (and just like humans, the rats would eat the filling first). A Princeton study found that, under certain circumstances, not only could rats become dependent on sugar, but this dependency correlated with several aspects of addiction, including craving, binging, and withdrawal. Medical addiction changes brain chemistry to cause binging, craving, withdrawal symptoms, and sensitization. Excess added sugar can do this too, through changes in the same pathways as addiction to amphetamines or alcohol. Sugar addiction could be an even harder habit to break, according to recent evidence about how added sugar affects our stress hormones. Sugar is also much more prevalent, available, and socially acceptable than amphetamines or alcohol, and so harder to avoid. There is an increasing body of research demonstrating that sugar can stimulate the brain's reward processing center in a manner that mimics what is seen with some recreational drugs. In certain individuals with certain predispositions, this could manifest as an addiction to sugary foods."

The World Health Organization (WHO) has been warning people to reduce their intake of "free sugars" to less than 10 percent of daily calories since 1989, saying that doing so can lower one's risk for being obese, overweight, or experiencing tooth decay. "Free sugars" include both the sugars naturally found in honey and fruit juice, and sugar added to food and drinks.

On food labels, added sugars include words such as glucose, corn syrup, brown sugar, dextrose, maltose, and sucrose, as well as many others. are Most of this comes from beverages, including energy drinks, alcoholic drinks, soda, fruit drinks, and sweetened coffee and teas. Other common sources are snacks. These don't just include obvious perpetrators, like brownies, cookies, doughnuts, and ice cream. There are large quantities of added sugar in bread, salad dressing, granola bars, and even fat-free yogurt. High-calorie sweeteners are in over 95 percent of granola bars, cereals, and sugar-sweetened beverages, most often in the form of corn syrup, sorghum, and cane sugar. Reducing sugar, especially concentrated sugars, not only limits the amount of sugars ingested but also makes fewer sweet foods seem sweeter.

Reference

Michaud, D.S., Liu, S., Giovannucci, E., et al., "Dietary Sugar, Glycemic Load, and Pancreatic Cancer Risk in a Prospective Study." Journal of the National Cancer Institute, 94(17), 2002, pages 1293-1300.

Medical professionals and researchers are trying to determine the best ways to thwart and treat chronic pain. If pain is due to inflammation, what and how much a person eats is an important part of the problem. Many conditions are associated with inflammation, including injury or infection, rheumatoid arthritis, inflammatory bowel disease, pelvic inflammatory disorder, Crohn's disease, colitis, atherosclerosis, diabetes, hepatitis, asthma, chronic obstructive pulmonary disease, vasculitis, autoimmune disorders, some cancers, sinusitis, and chronic periodontitis. While some types of pain can only be relieved by medical treatments, chronic pain due to inflammation can be improved by following a healthier diet. A reasonably healthy diet allows the body to better manage pain. Studies suggest that people who carry excess fat, particularly in the abdominal area, are at higher risk of developing low-grade inflammation throughout their bodies. That extra body fat plays a role in painful health problems such as fibromyalgia, chronic headaches, abdominal pain, pelvic pain, arthritis, and lower back pain.

Eating a high-fat diet activates cells that promote inflammation in the body's fatty tissue. That inflammation contributes to obesity and medical conditions associated with being overweight, including insulin resistance, diabetes, and heart disease. Red meat particularly processed red meat like cold cuts, sausages, and bacon is high in saturated fat and, when regularly consumed as part of a traditional American diet, has been linked to low-grade chronic inflammation as well as pain.

Many of the studies linking omega-3 fatty acids consumed from fatty fish like salmon and herring, fish oils, flaxseeds, and other sources to the reduction of inflammation and chronic pain have involved patients with arthritis and cardiovascular heart disease. At least one study also found that even when inflammation was controlled by medication, omega-3s helped reduce residual pain that was due to factors other than inflammation. These findings led researchers to conclude that omega-3 fatty acids may be beneficial in the early stages of rheumatoid arthritis, before inflammation intensifies. However, not all fatty acids are created equal and the ratio of omega-3 fatty acids to omega-6 fatty acids (from palm, soybean, rapeseed, and sunflower) also matters. A study of people with knee osteoarthritis whose diet was higher in omega-6 fats than omega-3 fats had more pain and more physical limitations than those who had a higher ratio of omega-3 fats to omega 6. This supports the theory that the balance of different fats in a diet from different sources is as important as the types and amount of fat that a person eats.

Eating a plant-based diet may hold the key to fighting inflammation, obesity, and conditions that lead to painful chronic disease. A traditional Mediterranean-style diet, when used to replace a traditional American diet, has been shown to reduce markers of chronic inflammation as well as lowering the risk of developing or dying from chronic diseases associated with inflammation. To help reduce inflammation, one should increase fiber in the diet, and improve one's overall health, and substitute high-protein plant foods such as legumes, nuts, and whole grains for some or all of the meat in the daily diet.

For centuries, practitioners of Chinese herbal medicine, Ayurvedic medicine, and other alternative and complementary forms of health care have long known the value of medical herbs and spices, including those that reduce pain and inflammation. More recently, scientists have confirmed the anti-inflammatory effects of herbs and spices such as turmeric, cinnamon, ginger, cayenne, sage, and rosemary and continue to study their role in fighting pain. For instance, compounds in ginger are particularly effective in the gastro-intestinal tract. Cinnamon has been shown to reduce the severity and duration of menstrual pain. Turmeric can reduce joint pain in rheumatoid arthritis, inhibit cancer cells, and slow the progression of diabetes-related disorders. Substances in rosemary have the potential to fight a variety of inflammatory diseases, bronchial asthma, peptic ulcer, and liver toxicity, and protect against cancer.

Some dietary changes may not be appropriate for some medical conditions. And because nutrients, herbs, and other substances in supplemental form can sometimes interfere with medical treatments, or cause problems of their own, it is also important for a patient to tell his or her health care providers what vitamins or supplements he or she is taking. Always consult with one's primary care physician before implementing the recommendations in this book.

References

Collins B, Hoffman J, Martinez K, et al. A polyphenol-rich fraction obtained from table grapes decreases adiposity, insulin resistance and markers of inflammation and impacts gut microbiota in high-fat-fed mice. The Journal of Nutritional Biochemistry. 2016; 31:150-165.

Okifuji A, Hare BD. The association between chronic pain and obesity. Journal of Pain Research. 2015; 8:399-408.

21. LABOR PAIN

For years, most health care practices have not allowed women to drink or eat anything but ice chips during labor. However, after advances in medical care and new research, some hospitals are changing their rules. Some hospitals now allow clear liquids. Healthy women with low-risk pregnancies should no longer need to fast during labor, according to a study by the American Society of Anesthesiologists. Doctors began requiring women to fast during labor after it was documented in the mid-20th century that pregnant women who were put under general anesthesia had an increased risk for

aspiration. Aspiration occurs when food or liquid is inhaled into the lungs. Pregnant women are at increased risk for aspiration because the enlarged uterus puts upward pressure on the stomach. Obviously, we don't want women to go through this, so it was decided that women should not eat or drink during labor. Ice chips were allowed because they would melt, but all other fluids would come through an IV. In a Cochrane review, researchers combined evidence from five trials involving a total of 3,103 women, in which women were randomly assigned to eat/drink or not during labor. All of the women were in active labor and at low risk of needing a Cesarean. They concluded that there is no harm or benefit in restricting low-risk women from consuming food and drink during labor.

In 2017, another review the researchers included all five studies from the Cochrane review and added five more, amounting to

3,982 participants. The authors found that the people laboring under less restrictive eating and drinking policies had shorter labors by about 16 minutes. There were no differences in any other health outcomes. Only one of the trials considered maternal satisfaction and found that more of the eating group participants reported satisfaction with their nourishment during labor compared to the women given sips of water only (97% versus 55%). There were no cases of aspiration in any of the trials; however, the study sizes were not large enough to determine how often this rare outcome truly occurs. Aspiration can happen when a person is put to sleep with an anesthetic. If they vomit stomach contents into their mouth while "sleeping" and these contents, go back down through the airway and cause aspiration pneumonitis.

The authors of the Cochrane review note that most women seem to naturally limit their intake as labor gets stronger. They concluded that low-risk women should have the right to choose whether or not they would like to eat and drink during labor. No trial has examined eating during labor in people who are at higher risk of needing Cesareans with general anesthesia. Researchers in Iran surveyed mothers on their perceptions of food and drink restrictions during labor. The first study interviewed 600 women and found an association between reported pain levels and environmental sources of stress, laboring people under stress experienced more pain. One of the greatest reported sources of stress was "restricted fluid intake." About half of first-time moms and 78% of moms who had given birth before mentioned this as a stressor.

In another study, researchers conducted in-depth interviews with 24 low-risk women after they had given birth, but before leaving the hospital. The women were in three different hospitals, demographically diverse, and all had healthy infants. The interview responses were grouped into common themes and coded for data analysis. One of the reoccurring responses was disappointment about restrictions on eating and drinking during labor. Women commented that they "felt out of energy," "had no more strength," and "felt hungry from going so long without eating."

The "Nothing by Mouth" policy during labor began in the 1940s, when women were given inhaled anesthetics (ether or chloroform in imprecise amounts) or Twilight Sleep (an injection of morphine and scopolamine that caused unconsciousness and no memory of the birth). Aspiration was more common than it is today. In 1946, Dr. Curtis Mendelson published the landmark study responsible for "Nothing by Mouth" policies. He found that people who had general anesthesia while giving birth could inhale stomach contents, which in rare cases could lead to severe lung disease or death. When Dr. Mendelson looked at 44,016 women who gave birth from 1932 to 1945, he found that aspiration occurred in 66 of those women (0.15% or 1 in 667). All of the people who experienced aspiration had a mixture of anesthesia gas, ether, and oxygen given to them through a mask during the delivery. There were two deaths in the study and both women went under general anesthesia without airway protection and aspirated solid food and died of suffocation on the delivery table. Mendelson concluded that aspirations are preventable and recommended replacing oral intake with IV fluids. Another review found that the people laboring under less-restrictive eating and drinking policies had shorter labors by about 16 minutes and no other differences in health outcomes. Only one of the trials in the review considered maternal satisfaction and found that more of the eating group participants reported satisfaction with their nourishment during labor compared to the women given sips of water only. Applesauce or Jell-O can provide the energy needed during delivery. Multigrain bread or crackers, whole-wheat pasta, brown rice, and oatmeal are good sources of fiber and offer carbohydrates that will provide energy during a long labor. These can often be combined with your protein source and create a nutritious meal. Healthy women who are not at risk for aspiration should ask their medical care providers (including their physician anesthesiologist and obstetrician) if eating a light meal during labor is safe for them. A light meal could include fruit, light soups, toast, light sandwiches (no large slices of meat), juice and water. Most women lose their appetites during very active labor, but can continue to drink fluids such as water and clear juices

References

1. Berry H. Feast or famine? Oral intake during labour: Current evidence and practice. British Journal of Midwifery. 1997;5(7):413–417
2. Hodnett ED. Pain and women's satisfaction with the experience of childbirth: a systematic review. Am J Obstet Gynecol 2002;186:S160–72.
3.

22. SUMMARY

Sweet tasting foods have been found to have an analgesic effect. Therefore, people might consume more sweet-tasting food when they feel pain. Patients eat more sweet-tasting food following a painful experience than a non-painful or a resource-depleting experience. These differences were not present for consumption of non-sweet food. Further, habitual self-control predicted consumption of sweet-tasting food when in pain, with those lower in self-control particularly likely to eat more. Results suggest that people do eat more sweet-tasting food when they feel pain, particularly if they are not in the habit of controlling their impulses. These findings have implications for health given rising rates of obesity and pain-related diagnoses.

Pain could impair one's choice because it alters the value assigned to sweet-tasting food. There is evidence that consumption of sweet-tasting food (i.e., high in sucrose), actually does impact the experience of pain. For example, consumption of sweet-tasting foods increases pain tolerance through endogenous opioid activity in the brain and opiate receptor antagonists (e.g., naloxone) can reduce the hedonic value of sweet-tasting foods. As a result of this connection between consumption of sweet-tasting foods and pain reduction the value assigned to foods high in sucrose might increase in conjunction with the experience of acute physical pain, with people enacting this heightened value by consuming more sweet-tasting food after pain experiences. Interestingly, evidence suggests that pain could increase consumption without altering self-reported liking of the stimuli. People demonstrate increased motivation to attain rewards during pain, but self-reports of liking are not changed, and after the experience of pain the typical relationship between self-reported liking of a food and consumption is disrupted.

Acute physical pain impairs in the sense that it results in increased consumption of sweet-tasting food. This finding may have important implications for public health, given that physical pain is a common daily occurrence and that there are many people living with chronic pain which is accompanied by periods of acute pain. If physical pain, an almost daily experience, increases consumption of sweet-tasting, frequently unhealthy, foods, there could be serious health and economic consequences. There is growing worldwide concern about obesity and related health problems, including diabetes, heart disease, and certain types of cancer, costing billions per year in lost productivity and health care.

Pain physiology involves complex immune, sensory, hormonal and inflammatory processes in the periphery, spinal cord, and brain. Repetitive nociceptive stimulation induces pathophysiological changes in the pain pathways leading to peripheral or central sensitization; hence, resulting in chronic pain in susceptible patients. Although evidence is limited, identifying risk factors and early multimodal approach and biopsychosocial assessment are reasonable steps to reduce the risk of developing chronic pain.

The previous mentioned information throughout this text reveals that changes in the valuation of pleasurable positive food can follow from a painful experience, as reflected by increased consumption. People do attempt to eat their pain away, likely based on previous experiences with certain foods having an analgesic effect after painful experiences. Given the availability of sweet-tasting foods, this increased consumption after pain has potentially deleterious consequences for health, especially for those with chronic pain conditions. However, the theme of this book is encouraging because multiple studies have been reported to date that with proper nutrition there is a significant probability that in some situations that chronic pain can be significantly reduced or in some cases even be eliminated. It is furthermore important for one to know that opioids decrease pain by exerting effects in the brain as well as the dorsal horn of the spinal cord. Numbing medications (lidocaine, bupivacaine) decrease pain impulses to the brain by inhibiting pain impulses at the posterior of the spinal cord. Topical anesthetics decrease pain impulses at the site of injury. Nutrition on the other hand can possibly decrease pain throughout the entire body in some cases and should be utilized in both acute and chronic pain conditions.

Good nutrition is often the first line of defense to avoid many diseases, including peripheral neuropathy. The best way to prevent peripheral neuropathy is to carefully manage any medical condition that puts you at risk. That means controlling your blood sugar level if you have diabetes or talking to your doctor about safe and effective treatments if you think you may have a problem with alcohol. Whether or not you have a medical condition, eat a healthy diet rich in fruits, vegetables, whole grains and lean protein. Keep a food diary so you are aware of what you're eating and to make sure you get all the nutrients you need each day to stay as healthy as possible. A diet rich in fish, nuts, whole grains, and fresh produce can be a part of a plan to maintain a healthy weight, which can reduce the effects of peripheral neuropathy as well. Food choices can increase or decrease inflammation. Chronic inflammation has been determined to be the cause of many chronic diseases, from autoimmune disorders like lupus, rheumatoid arthritis and cancer. Vinegar and cinnamon have been found to reduce increases in blood sugar by 20% to 30% and 6%, respectively. Vitamin D is known to decrease levels of inflammation. The chronic pain population, including those with fibromyalgia, is generally deficient in vitamin D. Pain patients without adequate vitamin D levels tend to stay on opioids twice as long and take twice as much of the drug as patients with appropriate vitamin D levels. Turmeric contains 6 identified NSAIDs.\ and may be helpful in decreasing inflammatory pain as well.

Opioid treatment has a profound effect on the endocrine–nutrition system, compounding the necessity of a pain diet. Weight gain may be profound, with some patients doubling their weight within a few years. Opioid use may cause blood sugar levels to be very unstable and may cause hypoglycemia. Opioids cause a "sugar desire effect" on opioid receptors. Consequently, the combination of severe chronic pain and opioid treatment can cause changes of glucose metabolism in patients and a desire to ingest primarily sugars and starches, with little protein or fat intake. Clinical observations of patients with chronic pain who require opioid treatment support the scientific research and the adverse effects of pain and opioids on the endocrine–nutrition systems. Pain patients with chronic pain report a gross deficiency of protein intake. It is recommended that pain practitioners take a dietary history for protein intake and examine the patient for muscle loss and weakness. Patients with pain may drink large amounts of sugar drinks and milk. A major element of the diet recommended here is stabilization of blood sugars.

A chronic pain diet should be based on high-protein intake. Endogenous pain relievers are protein derivatives. Amino acids enter the blood from the intestine and travel to locations in the liver, glands, and brain, where they are building blocks for compounds critical to pain relief. These include endorphin, dopamine, serotonin, and γ-aminobutyric acid (GABA). Insulin and thyroid hormones are derived from amino acids. The complaint of weakness by patients with severe pain may have many causes, but a lack of protein is one of them. Furthermore, the receptors to which pain-modulating neurotransmitters (endorphin, serotonin, and GABA) attach are protein moieties. A number of amino acids are required to build muscle. The amino acid proline is the major building block of collagen, which is essential for the development of cartilage and intervertebral discs.

References

Arnow B., Kenardy J., & Agras W. S. (1995). The Emotional Eating Scale: The development of a measure to assess coping with negative affect by eating. International Journal of Eating Disorders, 18, 79–90.

Darbor KE, Lench HC, Carter-Sowell AR (2016) Do People Eat the Pain Away? The Effects of Acute Physical Pain on

Subsequent Consumption of Sweet-Tasting Food. PLoS
ONE 11(11): e0166931 doi.

Gandhi W., Becker S. & Schweinhardt P. (2013). Pain
increases drive to obtain reward but does not affect
associated hedonic responses: A behavioral study in healthy
volunteers. European Journal of Pain, 17, 1093–1103.

Lewkowski M. D., Young S. N., Ghosh S., & Ditto B.
(2008). Effects of opioid blockade on the modulation of
pain and mood by sweet taste and blood pressure in young
adults. Pain, 135, 75–81. 10.1016/j.pain.2007.

Riva P., Wesselmann E. D., Wirth J. H., Carter-Sowell A.
R., & Williams K. D. (2014). When pain does not heal: The
common antecedents and consequences of chronic social
and physical pain. Basic and Applied Social
Psychology, 36, 329–346.

www.ingramcontent.com/pod-product-compliance
Lightning Source LLC
Chambersburg PA
CBHW051442250726
48655CB00001B/193